Nilufer Tarimci
C.Tuba Sengel Turk
Ulya Badilli

A novel approach for topical delivery of SLNs: Semisolid SLNs

AF141885

Nilufer Tarimci
C.Tuba Sengel Turk
Ulya Badilli

A novel approach for topical delivery of SLNs: Semisolid SLNs

LAP LAMBERT Academic Publishing

Impressum / Imprint
Bibliografische Information der Deutschen Nationalbibliothek: Die Deutsche Nationalbibliothek verzeichnet diese Publikation in der Deutschen Nationalbibliografie; detaillierte bibliografische Daten sind im Internet über http://dnb.d-nb.de abrufbar.
Alle in diesem Buch genannten Marken und Produktnamen unterliegen warenzeichen-, marken- oder patentrechtlichem Schutz bzw. sind Warenzeichen oder eingetragene Warenzeichen der jeweiligen Inhaber. Die Wiedergabe von Marken, Produktnamen, Gebrauchsnamen, Handelsnamen, Warenbezeichnungen u.s.w. in diesem Werk berechtigt auch ohne besondere Kennzeichnung nicht zu der Annahme, dass solche Namen im Sinne der Warenzeichen- und Markenschutzgesetzgebung als frei zu betrachten wären und daher von jedermann benutzt werden dürften.

Bibliographic information published by the Deutsche Nationalbibliothek: The Deutsche Nationalbibliothek lists this publication in the Deutsche Nationalbibliografie; detailed bibliographic data are available in the Internet at http://dnb.d-nb.de.
Any brand names and product names mentioned in this book are subject to trademark, brand or patent protection and are trademarks or registered trademarks of their respective holders. The use of brand names, product names, common names, trade names, product descriptions etc. even without a particular marking in this work is in no way to be construed to mean that such names may be regarded as unrestricted in respect of trademark and brand protection legislation and could thus be used by anyone.

Coverbild / Cover image: www.ingimage.com

Verlag / Publisher:
LAP LAMBERT Academic Publishing
ist ein Imprint der / is a trademark of
OmniScriptum GmbH & Co. KG
Heinrich-Böcking-Str. 6-8, 66121 Saarbrücken, Deutschland / Germany
Email: info@lap-publishing.com

Herstellung: siehe letzte Seite /
Printed at: see last page
ISBN: 978-3-659-77901-5

A NOVEL APPROACH FOR TOPICAL DELIVERY OF SLNs: SEMISOLID SLNs

Nilufer TARIMCI

Ankara University Faculty of Pharmacy

Department of Pharmaceutical Technology

Ankara/TURKEY

Ceyda Tuba SENGEL-TURK

Ankara University Faculty of Pharmacy

Department of Pharmaceutical Technology

Ankara/TURKEY

Ulya BADILLI

Ankara University Faculty of Pharmacy

Department of Pharmaceutical Technology

Ankara/TURKEY

PREFACE

Today's rapid technological improvements have significant implications for the pharmaceutical industry. The most significant developments during the past 50 years in that industry have been controlled release systems and targeted drug delivery. The impetus for research in these areas has been the ineffectiveness of conventional drugs in the current treatment of diseases.

The focus on drug delivery studies has shifted from the micro sized systems of the past to nano-sized systems today. The nano drug delivery methods and advantages of these systems in treatment of diseases attract attention of the researchers in the pharmaceutical formulation fields.

The nano delivery systems mainly consist of nano emulsions, polymeric and lipid nano particles and liposomes. Lipid nano particles are one of the colloid drug carrier systems and both solid lipid nanoparticles (SLNs) and nano structured lipid carriers (NLC) are well tolerated systems.

This book consists of three chapters. The first chapter provides general information on SLNs, their advantaged, and preparation methods, explains characterisations and stability of SLNs and further provides various application methods in treatment. In the second chapter, various applications of the SLNs, which are effective carrier systems for drugs and cosmetics, with the special focus on topical applications are investigated in detail. Other SLN research studies on active pharmaceutical ingredients (API) used commonly in dermatology also included in that chapter. The final chapter of the book explains semi solid SLNs as the novel dosage forms. The semi solid SLNs is a new approach in drug delivery with limited number of studies in the literature covering its properties and effects. In this chapter, preparation of semi solid SLNs and their structures are discussed and relevant research is evaluated.

This book is prepared by experienced researchers. We hope that it will serve as a useful resource for those interested in learning about lipid nanoparticles and the work of research groups studying them.

Ankara, 2015

Nilufer TARIMCI, PhD
Ulya BADILLI, PhD
Ceyda Tuba SENGEL-TURK, PhD

Table of Contents

CHAPTER 1

SOLID LIPID NANOPARTICLES: GENERAL INFORMATION

Ceyda Tuba SENGEL-TURK

Solid lipid nanoparticles (SLNs) are sub-micron sized colloidal particles composed of biodegradable lipids that are solidsat body temperature. A schematic illustration of an SLN is shown in Figure 1 (Lasa-Saracibar et al., 2012; Ekambaram et al., 2012). The first solid lipid nano-sized particles (called nanopellets) for peroral administration were prepared in 1980s by Speiser (1990) using a spray drying technique. In the 1990s, spherical lipid matrix sub-micron particles were developed by Müller et al. (1993), who used high pressure homogenisation methods to produce SLNs (Müller et al., 1993; Schwarz et al., 1994) and also by Gasco et al., who prepared SLNs using a warm microemulsion technique (Gasco et al, 1992; Gasco, 1993; 1997).

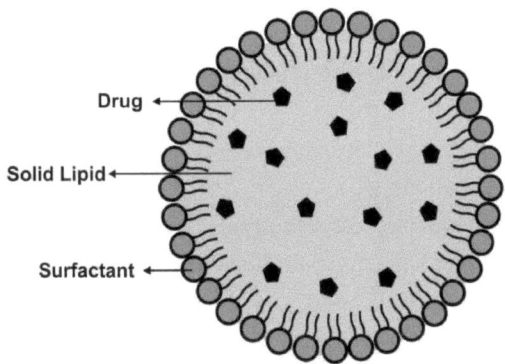

Figure 1. Structure of a solid lipid nanoparticle (SLN) (modified from Lohani et al., 2014).

The active compound is incorporated into a solid matrix structure, which creates difficulties for the diffusion of the active substance to the surface of the particles. The system consists of a solid lipid core matrix, into which lipophilic drug molecules can be solubilised. The lipid core is stabilised by various emulsifiers and the solid lipids provide the controlled release of the active agents from the particles. The lipid utilised in the preparation of the SLN formulations provides to have a low toxicity and high physical stability, when compared to other drug delivery systems such as liposomes (Sharma et al., 2011; Garud et al., 2012).

Major Advantages of SLNs

Sub-micron particles made from solid lipids are attracting major attention as novel colloidal drug carriers for application to other colloidal carriers such as liposomes, niosomes, nanoemulsions, nanosuspensions and polymeric nanoparticles. Some of the superior properties of SLNs over other carriers are listed in Table 1 (Mehnert and Mäder, 2001; Harde et al., 2011; Sharma et al., 2011; Garud et al., 2012; Jaafar-Maalej et al., 2012).

The most important advantages of the SLNs are the following (Cavalli et al., 1997; Schwarz and Mehnert, 1997; Freitas and Müller, 1998a; Zur Mühlen et al., 1998; Mehnert and Mäder, 2001; Wissing et al., 2004; Pandita et al., 2011; Battaglia & Gallarate, 2012):

- High drug loading of the entrapped drug molecule
- The excipients used in the production process of SLNs are non-toxic and biocompatible
- Both hydrophilic and hydrophobic active agents as well as the biotechnological therapeutics can be applied
- High storage and biological stability
- Possibility of prolonged or controlled drug release
- Capability of site-specific drug targeting
- Use of organic solvents is avoided in the SLN production process
- Possibility of lyophilisation
- Ease of sterilisation by autoclaving or gamma irradiation
- Ease of large-scale production
- High protection of active molecules against chemical degradation
- Ease of surface modification of SLN formulations with various coating agents
- Low manufacturing costs because the lipids used in SLN production are less expensive than synthetic polymers

Major Drawbacks of SLNs

Despite their advantages, SLN formulations have several major drawbacks (Battaglia & Gallarate, 2012; Araújo et al., 2013; Yadav et al., 2013):
- Polymorphic transitions during the storage period can result in drug leakage
- The physico-chemical properties of the entrapped drug molecule (especially hydrophilic substances) may results in insufficient drug loading
- SLN dispersions contain relatively high water content in their structures (70–99.9%)
- Different colloidal compositions/formations may be found in the dispersion medium
- Particle aggregation or growth may occur during long-term storage

Table 1. Important superior properties of solid lipid nanoparticles (SLNs) compared to other sub-micron colloidal drug delivery systems.

Important Parameters	Drug Delivery Systems					
	Liposomes	Niosomes	SLNs	Polymeric nanoparticles	Nanosuspensions	Nanoemulsions
Drug loading	Low to moderate	Moderate to high	High	Moderate	High	High
Drug targeting capability	Moderate	Moderate	Moderate	Moderate	Low	Low
Ability for hydrophilic drug incorporation	High	High	High	High	-	High
Ability for hydrophobic drug incorporation	High	High	High	High	High	High
Facility for gene delivery	Moderate	Moderate	Moderate	Moderate	-	Low
Suitability for oral administration	-	High	High	High	High	High
Suitability for parenteral application	High	high	High	High	High	High
Physiological stability	Low	Moderate	High	High	Moderate	Moderate
Storage stability	Low	Low	High	High	High	Moderate
Biocompatibility	High	High	High	Moderate	Moderate	High

8

Classification of the Main Excipients Used SLNs Production

The main ingredients presented in the formulations of the SLNs are the follows:

- Solid lipids
- Surfactants/Co-Surfactants
- Water

SLN formulations typically contain 0.1–30% solid lipid, which is dispersed in an aqueous phase stabilised with various surfactants. The lipids used in any of the SLN formulation are physiological components with Generally Recognised As Safe (GRAS) features. Partial glycerides, triglycerides, waxes, steroids and fatty acids are the main classes of lipids used in the SLN manufacturing process (Freitas and Müller, 1998b; Puglia & Bonina, 2012; Yadav et al., 2013).

Other important excipients involved in the production of lipid particles are the surfactants. These reduce the interfacial tension between the lipid and water phases and promote the formation of particles. Virtually all types of surfactants, varying in molecular weight and surface charge, have been utilised in stabilisinglipid dispersions. Generally, dispersion stabilisation is achieved by surfactants or the combination of surfactants/co-surfactants at 0.5–5 percent. Recent studies have confirmed that the combined use of co-surfactants with the surfactants is more efficient at preventing particle agglomeration during the SLN production process(Mehnert and Müller, 2001; Puglia and Bonina, 2012). The main surfactant types used in the SLN formulations are different type of lecithins, various kinds of poloxamers, polysorbates and bile salts. The administration route, especially for parenteral applications, is the major factor affecting the choice of surfactant type (Mehnert & Mäder, 2001; Wissing et al., 2004).

A summary of the main excipients commonly used in the SLN manufacturing process is given in Table 2.

Table 2. Classification of major excipients used for manufacturing of solid lipid nanoparticles (SLNs).

Kinds of Solid Lipid	References
Partial Glycerides	
Glyceryl monostearate (Geleol®, Imwitor®900)	Souto et al.(2005); Shah et al.(2007); Jensen et al. (2010)
Glyceryl palmitostearate (Precirol®ATO5)	Maia et al.(2000); Maia et al.(2002); Liu et al.(2007);Bhalekar et al.(2009)
Glyceryl behenate (Compritol®888ATO)	Jenning et al.(2000); Jenning et al.(2001); Pople & Singh (2006); Castro et al.(2007); Castro et al.(2011)
Triglycerides	

9

Trimyristin (Dynasan®114)	Wissing et al.(2001); Souto et al.(2005);Bhaskar et al.(2009); Pople & Singh (2010)
Tripalmitin (Dynasan®116)	Souto et al.(2004); Souto & Müller (2006); Souto & Müller (2007); Ruktanonchai et al.(2009); Jensen et al.(2011);
Tristearin (Dynasan®118)	Jain et al.(2010); Jensen et al.(2010); Nikolic et al.(2011)
Hydrogenated coco-glycerides (Softisan®142)	Jensen et al.(2010)
Hydrogenated palm oil (Softisan®154)	Nikolic et al.(2011)

Waxes

Cetyl palmitate (Cutina®CP, Precifac®ATO5)	Dingler et al.(1999); Jenning et al.(2001); Sznitowska et al. (2000); Wissing & Müller.(2002)
Carnauba wax	Mitri et al.(2011); Nikolic et al.(2011)
Beeswax	Nikolic et al.(2011); Zhang & Smith.(2011)

Steroids

Cholesterol	Zur Mühlen et al.(1998); Kuo & Wang (2014)

Hard Fat

Witepsol®E85	Uner et al. (2005)
Witepsol®H37	Sznitowska et al. (2000)
Suppocire®NA150	Padois et al.(2011)

Fatty Acids

Behenic acid	Cavalli et al.(1997)
Decanoic acid	Gasco et al.(1992)
Palmitic acid	Gasco et al.(1992)
Stearic acid	Iscan et al.(2005); Jain et al.(2005); Puglia et al.(2009); Trombino et al.(2009)

Types of Surfactants/Co-Surfactants
Lecithin

Soybean lecithin (Lipoid®S75, Lipoid®S100)	Maia et al.(2000); Jain et al.(2005); Liu et al.(2007)
Egg lecithin (Lipoid®E80)	Westesen et al.(1997)
Phosphatidylcholine (Epikuran®200, Phospholipon®80/H)	Grabnar et al.(2006); Shah et al.(2007); Fang et al.(2008); Padois et al.(2011)

Poloxamers

Poloxamer 188 (Lutrol®F68, Pluronic®F68)	Pople & Singh (2006);Souto & Müller (2006); Puglia et al.(2008); Ruktanonchai et al.(2009);
Poloxamer 407	Müller et al.(1996)
Poloxamine 908	Müller et al.(1996)

Polysorbates

Polysorbate 20 (Tween®20)	Iscan et al.(2005); Trombino et al.(2009)
Polysorbate 80 (Tween®80)	Wissing & Müller (2002); Jee et al.(2006); Liu et al.(2007); Sanna et al.(2007); Shah et al.(2007); Bhalekar et al.(2009); Passerini et al.(2009); Puglia et al.(2009); Jain et al.(2010); Jensen et al.(2010); Jensen et al.(2011);
Bile Salts	
Sodium cholate	Maia et al.(2002); Souto & Müller (2006)
Sodium glycocholate	Westesen et al.(1997); Bocca et al.,(1998); Cavalli et al.(1999)

Main SLN Manufacturing Techniques

Although various approaches are commonly used for the preparation of homogeneously dispersed SLN formulations, the basic production techniques can be explained as some variation of two main steps: the first step is the formation of an oil-in-water nano premulsion, and the second is the subsequent solidification of the aqueous dispersed phase. The main production techniques are as follows:

- High pressure homogenisation
    - Hot homogenisation
    - Cold homogenisation
- Microemulsion based method
- Solvent emulsification-evaporation method
- Solvent diffusion method
- Solvent injection method
- Double emulsion method
- High shear homogenisation and/orultrasonication technique
- Preparation by using membrane contactor
- Supercritical fluid technique

Details, advantages and disadvantages of each preparation techniques are as follows:

High pressure homogenisation

In recent years, among the differenttechniques available for production of SLNs, high pressure homogenisation has been considered the most effective manufacturing procedureby researchers for several reasons, including avoidance of the use of organic solvents, suitability for parenteral emulsion production, narrow particle size distribution, applicability to large-scale production and availability of homogenisation processes in industry (Müller et a., 2000; Mehnert & Mäder, 2001; Battaglia & Gallarate, 2012).High pressure homogenisers propel the fluid at high pressure (100-2000 bar) through a narrow hole a few microns in size. The liquid is expelled a very short distance at very high velocity(over 1000 km/h). The particles are broken up into smaller sizes by the turbulence and the cavitation of the system(Garud et al., 2012). This production technique is divided into two basic approaches according to the temperature used in the preparation process. Application at elevated temperatures is referred to as hot homogenisation and below room temperature is termed cold homogenisation (Wissing et al., 2004). Both approaches have the active compound dissolved into the lipid, which is melted at a temperature 5–10°C above its melting point. In the hot homogenisation approach, the melted lipid, includingthe active substance, is pre-emulsified into an aqueous emulsifier solution held at the same temperature as the lipid phase. The resulting pre-emulsion is homogenised using a high shear mixing homogeniser and the cooling of this hot oil/water (O/W) nanoemulsion leads to recrystallisation of the lipid and formation of the SLNs.

The high process temperatures used in this approach reduce the viscosity of the lipid phase and produce smaller-sized particles. However, the higher temperatures can cause degradation of highly temperature-sensitive drugs. The cold homogenisation method overcomes this drawback and is also used forhydrophilic drugs, which distribute into the aqueous phase during the hot homogenisation process, and for overcoming the recrystallisation difficulties associated with the nanoemulsion (Mehnert & Mäder, 2001; Jores et al., 2004). The cold method involves quick cooling of the mixture of the lipid melt and the active compound using liquid nitrogen or dry ice. The lipid in the solid structure is then ground to micron-sized particles. The obtained particles are then dispersed in a cold emulsifier solution and homogenised to break the micron sized particles into nano-sized solid lipid nanoparticles. This approach causes a broader size distribution and larger sized particles compared with the hot homogenisation approach (Müller et al., 2000; Wissing et al., 2004; Garud et al., 2012).

Microemulsion based method

Gasco et al. (1997) developed a new technique for producing SLNs and optimised the process. This method is based on the precipitation of the lipid phase by the addition of a microemulsion to a water phase and the formation of solid particles (Gasco, 1993; 1997). This production technique involves the preparation of a warm microemulsion composed of solid lipid (~10%), emulsifier (~15%) and co-emulsifier (~10%) by heating the lipids above their melting points and stirring them with the emulsifier and co-emulsifier to form a mixture. The resulting O/W microemulsion is dispersed in cold water, which precipitates the solid lipid nano-sized particles. The excess water is removed by lyophilisation or ultrafiltration (Cavalli et al., 1997; Battaglia& Gallarate, 2012).

Solvent emulsification-evaporation method

One major advantage of the emulsification-evaporation technique is that it avoids the use of heat during the production process. This then allows the loading of highly thermolabile drugs into the SLN formulations. This preparation technique is initiated by dissolving the lipid matrix material in a water-immiscible organic solvent, such as cyclohexane or chloroform. The resulting solution is then emulsified by high pressure homogenisation in an aqueous phase that includes various surfactants/co-surfactants. The organic solvent is then removed by evaporation and the lipid precipitates in the form of solid-state nanoparticles. The main drawback is the presence of organic solvent residues in the final product (Sjostrom & Bergenståhl, 1992; Cortesi et al., 2002).

Solvent diffusion method

The solvent diffusion technique is initiated by dissolving the lipid in a partially water miscible organic solvent, such as ethyl formate or benzyl alcohol. This solution is then emulsified in an aqueous surfactant solution at an elevated temperature. The organic solvent diffuses from the lipid phase to the aqueous phase after the addition of an excess amount of water, causing nano-sized solid lipid particles to precipitate. The obtained SLNs are then collected by centrifugation and freeze-dried (Quintanar-Guerrero et al., 2005).

Solvent injection method

Among the solvent-based production processes, the solvent injection technique is the most basic and the simplest. This method is based on the solubility of the lipid in a water miscible organic solvent such as acetone, ethanol or isopropanol and involves injection of this solution into an aqueous phase through a needle under gentle stirring. The solid lipid nano-sized particles are formed spontaneously by the precipitation of the lipid (Schubert & Müller-Goyman, 2003).

Double emulsion method

The double emulsion method is a manufacturing technology that allows the incorporation of the poorly-encapsulating, hydrophilic, active agents into SLNs. This production technique is based on the solvent emulsification-evaporation method and also consists of two steps. First, a w/o emulsion is produced by addition of a water phase containing the active substance to a melted lipid containing the surfactant and co-surfactant mixture. In the second step, the obtained emulsion is added to a second water system consisting of other surfactant and co-surfactant mixtures. The nano-sized solid lipid particles are successfully generated by cooling and obtained by ultra-filtration. The main disadvantage of this production method is that it forms large particles (Morel et al., 1998).

Electrospraying

Electrospraying is a novel technology only recently applied to SLN production (Trotta et al., 2010; Cavalli et al., 2011). This technology is a one-step production process which provides micro- or nano-sized particles with a narrow size distribution. The system is based on the capability of an electric field to create a deformation on the interface of a droplet. Application of an electric field to a droplet causes the formation of an electrostatic force inside the droplet that can exceed the cohesive force of the droplet. In this way, the droplet can be broken up into smaller ones in the nano size range. Solid lipid particles can be formed during the evaporation of a solvent from the droplet as it travels through an electrical field. The suitability of this technique for SLN production was first examined by Trotta et al. (2010), in terms of various physicochemical characteristics of the particles,who showed that this technology could be successfully applied for the production of tamoxifen-loaded SLN formulations (Trotta et al., 2010).

High shear homogenisation and/or ultrasonication technique

High-shear homogenisation and ultrasound processes are alternative methods for the preparation of SLNs and are often used in conjunction. The basic advantages of these technologies are the ease of handling and freedom from organic solvent use. However, the main disadvantages are the low quality of the dispersion and risk of metallic contamination by the use of ultrasound technology (Garud et al., 2012; Jaafar-Maalej et al., 2012).

Preparation using a membrane contactor

Membrane contactor technology allows the large-scale production of SLNs. This method begins by heating the lipid to a temperature above its meting point, followed by pressing the melted lipid through membrane pores to form small droplets. SLNs are obtained after cooling the preparation to room temperature. The temperatures of the phases, the cross-flow velocity of the aqueous phase, the membrane pore size and the pressure of the lipid phase are the important factors that affect the quality of the final product when using this technology (Charcosset et al., 2005).

Supercritical fluid technique

Another manufacturing process applied for the production of SLNs is supercritical fluid technology. In this approach, a liquid is termed supercritical when its temperature and pressure surpass their own critical values. Carbon dioxide is the most common liquid used as a supercritical fluid due to its non-toxicity and low manufacturing cost. The major superior properties of this technology are its avoidance of the use of organic solvents in the production process and the generation of the particles in a dry powder form (Battaglia & Gallarate, 2012; Garud et al., 2012).

Characterisation of SLNs

Performing quality control on SLN formulations requires the application of appropriate instrumental characterisation techniques. However, characterisation of SLN formulations is a critical problem due to their dynamic structure and the complexity and the submicron size of the developed systems. The most important features of the SLNs include the following: drug loading and entrapment efficiency; particle size and size distribution; surface charge and shape features; crystal structure and polymorphic behaviour; drug release profiles and mechanisms; co-existence of additional colloidal structures, such as liposomes and micelles; rheological, adhesive and permeability properties; and cytotoxicity and cell uptake capabilities. Different instrumental techniques are available for determining these physicochemical and biological characteristics of the SLNs. The main properties are listed in Table 3.

Table 3. Summary of the major techniques used for the determination of the physicochemical and biological characteristics of solid lipid nanoparticle (SLN) formulations.

Characteristics	Techniques used for characterisation	References
Drug loading and incorporation efficiency	Dialysis; separation techniques such as membrane filtration, ultracentrifugation and gel permeation chromatography.	Lv et al., 2009; Pandita et al., 2011; Battaglia & Gallarate, 2012; Yadav et al., 2013
	Analytical techniques,such asultra-violet spectrophotometry (UV); high-performance liquid chromatography (HPLC); and spectrofluorophotometry, can be used to determine drug amounts.	
Particle size and size distribution	Photon correlation spectroscopy (PCS); Static light scattering (SLS)/Fraunhofer diffraction; Laser diffraction (LD); Scanning electron microscopy (SEM); Transmission electron microscopy (TEM); Atomic force microscopy (AFM); Field-flow fractionation (FFF); Packed column hydrodynamic (PCH); Size exclusion chromatography (SEC).	Freitas & Müller, 1998b; Mehnert & Mäder, 2001; Jores et al., 2004; Bhaskar et al., 2009; Elnaggar et al., 2011; Garud et al., 2012; Lasa-Saracibar et al., 2012; Patil et al., 2013; Yadav et al., 2013
Surface charge	Zeta potential by PCS; Laser droplet anemometry.	Schwarz & Mehnert, 1997; Freitas & Müller, 1998a; Lasa-Saracibar et al., 2012;

Morphology	Scanning electron microscopy (SEM); Transmission electron microscopy (TEM); Atomic force microscopy (AFM); Confocal laser scanning microscopy (CSLM); Fluorescence microscopy.	Cavalli et al., 1997; Mehnert & Mäder, 2001; Bhaskar et al., 2009; Pandita et al., 2011; Garud et al., 2012; Kuo & Wang, 2014.
Drug release	Separation by filtration or ultracentrifugation; Dialysis bag diffusion technique; Franz-type diffusion cell.	Sharma et al., 2011; Ekambaram et al., 2012; Elnaggar et al., 2011; Lasa-Saracibar et al., 2012;
Crystal structure analysis and polymorphic behaviour	Differential scanning calorimetry (DSC); X-ray diffraction (XRD); Cryo-electron microscopy; Raman spectroscopy; Fourier transform infrared spectroscopy (FTIR).	Mehnert & Mäder, 2001; Bunjes et al., 2003; Bunjes et al., 2007; Garud et al., 2012; Yadav et al., 2013.
Co-existence of additional forms	Nuclear magnetic resonance (NMR); Electron spin resonance (ESR).	Morel et al., 1998; Müller et al., 2000; Mehnert & Mäder, 2001; Patil et al., 2013; Yadav et al., 2013.
Rheological properties	Rheometer	Badilli et al., 2014; Bhaskar et al., 2009
Adhesive activity	Textural profile analysis (TPA)	Karavana et al., 2012; Amasya G, 2014.
Occlusive properties	In vitro occlusion test.	Müller et al., 2002
Permeability features	Franz-type diffusion cell using appropriate animal skin membrane; Cell culture studies with co-culture models	Cecchelli et al., 1999; Bhaskar et al., 2009; Lv et al., 2009; Elnaggar et al., 2011; Kuo & Wang, 2014.
Cell viability and cytotoxicity	MTT cell viability assay.	Ridolfi et al., 2011; Barbosa et al., 2013
In vitro cellular uptake	HPLC; Confocal laser scanning microscopy (CSLM); Fluorescence.	Amasya G, 2014, Kuo & Wang, 2014.

MTT: 3-(4,5-dimethylthiazol-2-yl)-2,5-diphenyltetrazolium bromide

These techniques have all been described and scrutinised in the literature. However, the underlying foundations of these characterisation techniques are basic and similar to methods used for other nano-sized particles. Therefore, researchers are in agreement with the different incorporation models and drug release principles specific to SLNs that distinguish the SLNs from other submicron-sized drug delivery systems.

Incorporation Models of Drug Molecules into SLNs

Several factors affect the entrapment efficiency of an active compound into the SLN structure (Müller et al., 2000; Müller et al., 2002; Üner and Yener, 2007). These are:
- polymorphic form of the lipid material,
- physico-chemical nature of the solid lipid matrix used in the formulation
- solubility of the model compound into the melted lipid matrix,
- miscibility of the model compound and the lipid melt.

Three basic drug incorporation models proposed for the loading of the active ingredients into SLNs areshown in Figure 2.

I.   Solid solution model
II.   Active compound-enriched core model
III. Active compound -enriched shell model

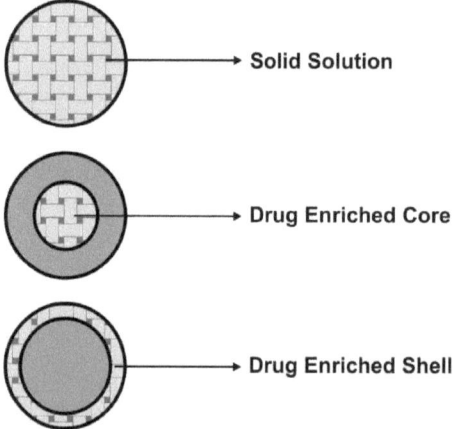

Figure 2. Types of drug incorporation models for solid lipid nanoparticle (SLN) formulations (modified from Müller et al., 2002).

The state of the active compound within the SLN structure is a function of the formulation ingredients and the preparation method. In the solid solution model, preparation of SLNs with a cold homogenisation technique results in dispersion or dissolution of the active ingredient at molecular level within the lipid matrix. The final SLN products with homogenous structures are formed by high mechanical fracturing during the manufacturing process. Similar matrix formation mechanisms can be observed in homogeneous dispersions of active ingredient in lipid droplets and in production methods that use hot homogenisation techniques. The solid solution entrapment model is characterised by a strong interaction between the active ingredient and the lipid material (Schwarz 1995, Zur Mühlen et al, 1998).

The second type of drug incorporation model for SLNs, the drug enriched core model, involves the formation of a core enriched with active agent during the cooling process of the nano droplets to generate the solid nanoparticles. The active compound, which is dissolved into the lipid melt at or close to its saturation solubility,becomes supersaturated during the cooling period and precipitates before the recrystallisation of the lipid. This means that the active substance is precipitated earlier than the lipid, which leads to recrystallisation of the lipid melt to form a lipid shell surrounding the active agent. The drug-free lipid shell structure gives a membrane-controlled release profile to the entrapped active agents based on Fick's law of diffusion (Müller et al., 2000; Müller et al., 2002).

The third type of drug incorporation models for SLNs, the drug enriched shell model, involves the formation of an outer shell enriched with the active compound during the liquid to solid phase separation of the lipid droplets that occurs during the cooling process. The lipid material can be precipitated first in this process to form a lipid core—the reverse of the second model type. This drug enriched shell structure allows a very fast drug release from the developed SLNs. This release profile can be suitable and also highly preferred for topical applications of a drug substance to provide an increased drug penetration (Müller et al., 2002; Wissing et al., 2004).

General Principles of Drug Release from SLNs

Some basic strategies have been proposed to explain the mechanisms underlying drug release from SLNs. The relevant parameters are the following (Zur Mühlen et al., 1998; Zur Mühlen & Mehnert, 1998; Mehnert & Müller, 2001; Müller et al., 2002; Wissing et al., 2004; Üner et al., 2007):

- A relationship exists between the production temperature applied during the production process and the drug release profile from the SLNs, depending on the preferred preparation technique. Many different researchers have demonstrated that drugs are usually released from SLNs in a biphasic manner: an initial burst release, followed by a prolonged release. However, increasing the production temperature of a hot homogenisation technique for the preparation of SLNs caused a decrease in the drug release from the SLNs; while a cold homogenisation technique showed no effect of the production temperature (Zur Mühlen et al., 1998; Mehnert & Müller, 2001; Müller et al., 2002).

- The incorporation of the active ingredient substantially affects the release pattern of the drug. As discussed above, this situation is related to the technique used for the preparation of the SLNs and the composition of the SLN formulation. The cold homogenisation method, as a production technique,uses the solid solution model and the active compounds are molecularly dispersed within the lipid phase of the system. The limited mobility of the drug moleculeslocated in the lipid matrix results in extension of drug release over several weeks. For the active compound-enriched core model, where the active compounds are surrounded by a membrane of lipids, membrane control becomes the main factor affecting the release of the active compound and Fick's law diffusion is the major mechanism that governs the drug release. Conversely, for the active compound-enriched shell model, a burst effect is seen during the initial minutes ofrelease experiments due to the high degree of localisation of the SLNs at the particle surface (Zur Mühlen & Mehnert, 1998; Müller et al., 2002).

- An inverse relationship is obtained between the partition coefficient of the active compound and the release profile of the drug from the system. A higher partition coefficient of the active ingredients leads to slower drug release from the developed SLN formulations (Zur Mühlen et al., 1998).

- Particle size is crucial to the drug release behaviour and directly affects the drug release rate. Lower surface area which is a result of bigger nano-sized particles reduced thedrug release (Zur Mühlen et al., 1998).

- Crystallisation behaviour of the lipid and the low mobility of the active compound lead to slow drug release from SLNs. An opposite relationship exists between the mobility potential of the active ingredient and the degree of crystallisation of the lipid. Zur Mühlen et al. (1998) concluded from their research that a retardationof recrystallisation of the lipid during the production process increased with decreasing concentrations of lipid and increasing amounts of emulsifier.

- Another major factor affecting the drug release pattern from SLNs is the emulsifier concentration. During the preparation process by the hot homogenisation technique, the active agent partitions from the liquid phase to the water phase and a higher emulsifier concentration leads to an increase in the saturation solubility of the active compound in the aqueous phase. During the cooling process, due to the decrease in temperature of the aqueous dispersion of the system, the solubility of the active agent in the aqueous phase is also reduced, and, as expected, the lipid recrystallises before the precipitation of the drug. This situation leads to the accumulation of the active ingredient on the surface of the particles. Therefore, higher emulsifier concentrations increase the burst release of the drug (Müller et al., 2000).

Stability Issues of SLNs

The changes in physicochemical characteristics of SLN dispersions during prolonged storage periods can be evaluated by monitoring their alterations in terms of the drug loading, particle size and size distribution, surface charge, drug-excipient interactions, appearance, lipid crystallisation, and viscosity as a function of time (Mehnert & Mäder, 2001; Wissing et al., 2004; Radomska-Soukharev, 2007). Effects of external factors such as light and temperature on the physical stability of the SLNs could be particularly important for long-term stability (Müller et al., 2002; Sharma et al., 2011, Ekambaram et al., 2012). Several researchers have stated that the physical their developed SLN formulations, when stored as aqueous dispersions,were stable for usually more than one year (Westesen et al., 1997; Westesen, 2000; Radomska-Soukharev, 2007), Müller et al. (2002) showed a stability of up to three years for SLNs prepared using Precirol®ATO5 or Compritol®888ATO as lipids.

The mean particle size of the SLN dispersion remained stable between 160 and 220 nm for three years at 4°C (Wissing et al., 2004). Freitas and Müller (1998a, b) evaluated the effects of light and temperature on the physical stability of aqueousSLN dispersionsprepared with Compritol®888ATO and Pluronic®F68 as lipid and emulsifier, respectively. They concluded that artificial light causedgelation of the system and growth in the particlesize within 7 days ofstorage, whereas a similar response took 3 months in daylight. In darkness, the particles started to grow in size after 4 months of storage.

Examination of the influence of the storage temperature on the particle size of the SLN dispersions revealed that the particle size increased swiftly at elevated temperatures but remained stable during 6 months of storage at 4°C (Freitas & Müller, 1998a). Despite the labile structure seen in aqueousSLN dispersions, SLN formulations can also be stored as dry powder forms. Aqueous SLN dispersions possess long term stability of up to 3 years, but prolonged long-term stability is required, especially for parenteral applications, and this can only be achieved by conversion to a dry powder form. Aqueous SLN dispersions can be converted into dry forms using several drying methods, such as spray-drying or lyophilisation techniques. The dry powder form could be more favourable for the SLN formulations containing active compounds which are quite sensitive to hydrolysis or to external factors such as light or elevated temperatures (Freitas & Müller, 1998b; Wissing et al., 2004).

Application Routes of the SLNs

SLNs can be applied by various administration routes, as described as follows:

Oral administration

The oral route is preferred for enhancing the bioavailability of the active compounds. In this case, SLNs act by protecting the agents against the microbacterial environment of the gastrointestinal tract and by improvingtransport through intestinal epithelial layer (Müller et al., 1996). Several antitubercular active agents, such as pyrazinamide, rifampicin and isoniazid, have been incorporated into SLN formulations that were developed and used for the therapy to improve patient compliance and reduce side effects by decreasing the dosage frequency (Pandey et al., 2005a and 2005b). Yang et al. (1999a, b) investigated the body distribution profile of camptothecin-loaded SLN formulations after oral administration of SLNs formed using soybean lecithin and stearic acid as lipid matrix materials and Poloxamer 188 as an emulsifier. The obtained SLNs were 197 nm in size with a -69 mV zeta potential value. Entrapment efficiency of the camptothecin into this SLN formulation was 99.6%. Measurement of plasma levels of the camptothecin after SLN administration showed that incorporation of the active compound into SLNs prevented the hydrolysis of the drug after oral administration. These researchersconcluded that SLN formulationsare very suitable drug delivery systems for the oral application of lipophilic agents such as camptothecin (Yang et al., 1999b).

Parenteral administration

Parenteral application of SLNs is preferred for site-specific targeting ofdrugs by the attachment of desired specific ligands and/or the delivery of poorly water-soluble compounds. SLN formulations are very convenient systems for achieving systemic delivery of the drugs because the lipid materials of the SLN systems are well-tolerated and physiologically compatible ingredients. SLN formulations also have excellent physical stability after sterilisation processesrequired for parenteral preparations. Particles of several colloidal systems injected intravenouslyare mostly cleared from the blood circulation by macrophages of the liver and the spleen. Hydrophobic coatingson the SLNs can protect the particles from macrophagic uptake,thereby improving the treatment (Müller et al., 2000; Wissing et al., 2004). Fundarò et al. (2000) prepared doxorubicin-loaded stealth and non-stealth SLNs and investigated their pharmacokinetics and tissue distribution after invivo administration to rats. After the intravenous administration of the SLNs, the plasma levels of doxorubicin were increased and prolonged. This research surprisingly showed that both stealth and non-stealth SLNs displayed lower and similar uptake by the liver and spleen macrophages (Fundarò et al., 2000).

Another parenteral application aim of SLNs is brain targeting. Yang et al. (1999a) studied the body distribution profile and the targeting effect to the brain of camptothecin-loaded SLN formulations after intravenous administration to mice. SLNs were produced using a high pressure homogenisation technique and Poloxamer 188, soybean lecithin and stearic acid were used as the emulsifier and the lipids, respectively. The authors found that SLN formulations resulted in increased drug uptake into the brain.

Ocular application

SLNs have improved the bioavailability of drugs when used in ocular applications. The muco-adhesive properties of the SLN formulations enhance the interaction between the particle surface and the ocular mucosa; thereby prolonging the corneal contact time of the active agent (Başaran et al., 2010). To date, many hydrophobic active agents, such as pilocarpine, cyclosporine-A, tobramycin andvitamin A, have been successfully entrapped into SLN formulations for ocular drug delivery. Topical application of SLNs was confirmed to enhance the transfer of the active compound into the aqueous humour (Gökce et al., 2008). Sandri et al.(2010) evaluated cyclosporine-A loaded SLN formulations associated with chitosan as carriers for ocular delivery through corneal cells. The permeation and penetration characteristics of the developed formulations were evaluated in in vivo cell culture and ex vivo excised pig cornea experiments. The chitosan-associated SLN formulations of cyclosporine A enhanced the penetration and permeation of the drug in both ex vivo and in vitro models. Another research group studied the in vivo corneal efficiency of topical cyclosporine-A-containing SLN formulations in rabbit eyes (Gökçe et al., 2009). They concluded that cyclosporine-A concentration reached therapeutic levels in the aqueous humour of the rabbit eyes 8 hours after application.

Nasal administration

The nasal route is a suitable alternative drug administration route because it provides rapid adsorption and fast onset of the drug action. It also protects labile drugs like proteins and peptides against the degradation processes occurring in the gastrointestinal channel. It is a promising disjunctive route for brain targeting of many active compounds, such as risperidone, methotrexate and 5-fluorouracil (Patel et al., 2011; Masserini, 2013; Van Woensel et al., 2013). Singh et al. (2012) incorporated alprazolam into SLN formulations and evaluated their targeting efficiency as drug carrier systems to brain through nose and their biodistribution profile in male Wistar rats after intranasal delivery. Gamma scintigraphy imaging studies were performed on New Zealand rabbits by tagging the formulation with radioactive ^{99m}Tc. These researchers found that the SLN structure protected alprazolam from chemical and/or biological degradation. This research revealed that alprazolam could be effectively and promptly transported to the brain via intranasal administration by crossing the blood brain barrier.

Rectal application

Many therapeutic situations require a rapid pharmacological response and rectal application is preferred in these cases. The therapeutic response and efficacy of the drugs applied via a rectal route are higher when compared withdrugs given intramuscularly or orally. Only a few studies have been published on the rectal administration of SLNs (Sznitowska et al., 2000; Sznitowska et al., 2001). Sznitowska et al. (2000) encapsulated diazepam into an SLN formulation for rectal delivery. The SLNs were prepared by a high pressure homogenisation technique using Witepsol®H37 as the main lipid in the formulation and lecithin as the emulsifier. Diazepam-loaded SLN formulations were successfully prepared and the researchers conducted another study in 2001 as a continuation of this work. The diazepam-incorporated SLN formulations were administered rectally to provide a rapid therapeutic response. They evaluated the bioavailability performance of the developed SLN dispersions in rabbits and declared that the lipid matrix used, which was solid in nature at body temperature, was not suitable for the rectal delivery of diazepam via SLNs.

Pulmonary delivery

Lungs are important sites for targeting and/or delivering drugs due to their large surface area for absorption. SLN aerosol systems are accepted as a new and upcoming research area for enhancement of drug bioavailability by pulmonary delivery (Üner &Yener, 2007; Jaafar-Maalej et al., 2012). Many drugs, such as rifampicin, isoniazid, pyrazinamide (Jaafar-Maalej et al., 2012), insulin (Liu et al., 2008), epirubicin (Hu et al., 2010) and amikacin (Ghaffari et al., 2011), have been formulated as SLNs for pulmonary delivery. Hu et al. (2010) evaluated the antineoplastic activity of epirubicin-loaded SLN formulations against lung cancer. The SLNs were produced as an inhalable system and their in vitro pulmonary deposition was determined. In vivo pharmacokinetic profile studies in rats showed that the inhaled drug concentration of epirubicin was much higher than that in the plasma when SLN formulations were applied via an inhalation route.

Dermal application

The advantages of dermal application of SLNs and examples of research covering these applications will be reviewed in detail in Chapter 2.

REFERENCES

Araújo, D.R., Silva, D.C., Barbosa, R.M., Franz-Montan, M., Cereda, C.M.S., Padula, C., Santi, P., Paula, E. Strategies for delivering local anesthetics to the skin: focus on liposomes, solid lipid nanoparticles, hydrogels and patches.*Expert Opin. Drug Deliv.,*10(11): 1551-1563, 2013.

Amasya, G. Quality by design studies and evaluation of lipid nanoparticles containing 5-fluorouracil in the treatment of skin cancers. Ph.D. Thesis, Ankara University, 2014.

Badilli, U., Sengel-Turk, C.T., Onay-Besikci, A., Tarimci, N.Development of etofenamate-loaded semisolid SLN dispersions and evaluation of anti-inflammatory activity for topical application. *Curr.Drug Deliv.,*12(2): 200-209, 2015.

Barbosa, R.M., de Silva, C.M.G., Bella, T.S., de Araújo, D.R., Marcato, P.D., Durán, N., de Paula, E. Cytotoxicity of solid lipid nanoparticles and nanostructured lipid carriers containing the local anesthetic dibucaine designed for topical application. *J. Physics,* 429: 012035, 2013.

Başaran, E., Demirel, M., Sırmagül, B., Yazan, Y. Cyclosporine A-incorporated cationic solid lipid nanoparticles for ocular delivery. *J. Microencapsul.,* 27: 37-47, 2010.

Battaglia, L. & Gallarate, M. Lipid nanoparticles: state of the art, new preparatipon methods and challenges in drug delivery.*Expert Opin. Drug Deliv.,*9(5): 497-508, 2012.

Bhalekar, M.R., Pokharkar, V., Madgulkar, A., Patil, N., Patil, N. Preparation and evaluation of miconazole nitrate-loaded solid lipid nanoparticles for topical delivery. *AAPS PharmSciTech,* 10: 289-296, 2009.

Bhaskar, K., Anbu, J., Ravichandiran, V., Venkateswarlu, V., Rao, Y.M. Lipid nanoparticles for transdermal delivery of flurbiprofen: formulation, in vitro, ex vivo and in vivo studies. *Lipids Health Dis.,*8: 6,2009.

Bocca, C., Caputo, O., Cavalli, R., Gabriel, L., Miglietta, A., Gasco, M.R. Phagozytic uptake of fluorescent stealth and non-stealth solid lipid nanoparticles. *Int. J. Pharm.,* 175: 185-193, 1998.

Bunjes, H., Koch, M.H., Westesen, K. Influence of emulsifiers on the crystallization of solid lipid nanoparticles. *J. Pharm. Sci.,* 92: 1509-1520, 2003.

Bunjes, H., Steiniger, F., Richter, W. Visualizing the structure of triglyceride nanopartciles in different crystal modifications. *Langmuir,* 23: 4005-4011, 2007.

Castro, G.A.,Orefice, R.L., Vilela, J.M.C., Andrade, M.S., Ferreira, L.A. Development of a new solid lipid nanoparticle formulation containing retinoic acid for topical treatment of acne. *J. Microencapsul.,* 24: 395-407, 2007.

Castro, G.A., Oliveira, C.A., Mahecha, G.A.B., et al. Comedolytic effect and reduced skin irritation of a new formulation of all-trans retinoic acid-loaded solid lipid nanoparticles for topical treatment of acne. *Arch. Dermatol. Res.,* 303: 513-520, 2011.

Cavalli, R., Caputo, O., Carlotti, M.E., Trotta, M., Scarnecchia, C., Gasco, M.R. Sterilization and freeze-drying of drug-free and drug-loaded solid lipid nanoparticles. *Int. J. Pharm.,* 148: 47-54, 1997.

Cavalli, R., Bocca, C.,Miglietta, A.,Caputo, O.,Gasco, M.R. Albumin adsorption on stealth and non-stealth solid lipid nanoparticles. *S.T.P. Pharma Sci.,* 9: 183-189, 1999.

Cavalli, R.,Bisazza, A., Bussano, R., Trotta, M., Civra, A., Lembo, D., Ranucci, E., Ferruti, P. Poly(amidoamine)-cholesterol conjugate nanoparticlesobtained by electrospraying as novel tamoxifen delivery system.*J. Drug Deliv.,*Volume 2011, Article ID 587604, 2011.

Cecchelli, R., Dehouck,B., Descamps, L., Fenart, L., Buee-Scherrer, V., Duhem, C., Lundquist, S., Rentfel, M., Torpier, G., Dehouck, M.P. In vitro model for evaluating drug transport across theblood–brain barrier.*Adv. Drug Deliv. Rev.,*36: 165–178,1999.

Charcosset, C., El-Harati, A., Fessi, H. Preparation of solid lipid nanoparticles using a membrane contactor. *J. Control. Release*, 108: 112-120, 2005.

Cortesi, R., Esposito, E., Luca, G., Nastruzzi, C. Production of lipospheres ascarriers for bioactive compounds. *Biomaterials*, 23:2283–2294, 2002.

Dingler, A., Blum, R.P., Niehus, H., Müller, R.H., Gohla, S. Solid lipid nanoparticles (SLN/Lipopearls). A pharmaceutical and cosmetic carrier forthe application of vitamin E in dermal products. *J. Microencapsul.,* 16: 751-767, 1999.

Ekambaram, P., Sathalı, A.A.H., Priyanka, K. Solid lipid nanoparticles: a review. *Sci. Revs. Chem. Commun.,*2(1): 80-102, 2012.

Elnaggar, Y.S.R., El-Massik, M.A., Abdallah, O.Y. Fabrication, appraisal, and transdermal permeationof sildenafil citrate-loaded nanostructured lipidcarriers versus solid lipid nanoparticles. *Int. J. Nanomed.,* 6: 3195-3205, 2011.

Fang, J.Y., Fang, C.L., Liu, C.H., Su, Y.H. Lipid nanoparticles as vehicles for topical psoralen delivery: solid lipid nanoparticles (SLN) versus nanostructured lipid carriers (NLC).*Eur. J. Pharm. Biopharm.,* 70: 633-640, 2008.

Freitas, C. & Müller, R.H. Effect of light and temperature on zeta potential and physical stability in solid lipid nanoparticles (SLN™) dispersions.*Int. J. Pharm.,* 168: 221-229, 1998a.

Freitas, C. & Müller, R.H. Spray-drying of solid lipid nanoparticles.*Eur. J. Pharm. Biopharm.,* 46: 145-151, 1998b.

Fundarò, A., Cavalli, R., Bargoni, A., Vighetto, D., Zara, G.P., Gasco, M.R. Nonstealth and stealth solid lipid nanospheres carrying doxorubicin: pharmacokinetics and tissue distribution after i.v. administration to rats. *Pharm. Res.,*42: 337-343, 2000.

Garud, A., Singh, D., Garud, N. Solid lipid nanopartciles (SLN): Method, characterization and applications. *Int. Cur. Pharmaceutic. J.,* 1(11): 384-393, 2012.

Gasco, M.R., Cavalli, R., Carlotti, M.E. Timolol in liphospheres. *Pharmazie,* 47: 119-121, 1992.

Gasco, M.R. Method for producing solid lipid microspheres having a narrow size distribution. *US*188837, 1993.

Gasco, M.R. Solid lipid nanospheres from warm microemulsions. *Pharm. Tech. Eur.,*9: 52-58, 1997.

Ghaffari, S., Varshosaz, J., Saadat, A., Atyabi, F. Stability and antimicrobial effect of amikacin-loaded solid lipid nanoparticles. *Int. J. Nanomedicine,* 6: 35-43, 2011.

Grabnar, P.A., Zajc, N., Kristl, J. Improvement of ascorbyl palmitate stability in lipid nanoparticle dispersions for dermal use. *J. Drug Deliv. Sci. Technol.,* 16: 443-448, 2006.

Gökçe, E.H., Sandri, G., Bonferoni, M.C., Rossi, S., Ferrari, F., Güneri, T., Caramella, C. Cyclosporine A-loaded SLNs: evaluation of cellular uptake and corneal cytotozicity. *Int. J. Pharm.,* 364: 76-86, 2008.

Gökçe, E.H., Sandri, G., Eğrilmez, S., Bonferoni, M.C., Güneri, T., Caramella, C. Cyclosporine A-loaded solid lipid nanoparticles: ocular tolerance and in vivo drug release in rabbit eyes. *Curr. Eye Res.,* 34: 996-1003, 2009.

Harde, H., Das, M., Jain, S. Solid lipid nanoparticles: an oral bioavailability enhancer vehicle. *Expert Opin. Drug Deliv.,* 8(11): 1407-1424, 2011.

Hu, L., Jia, Y., Wen, D. Preparation and characterization of solid lipid nanoparticles loaded with epirubicin for pulmonary delivery. *Pharmazie,* 65: 585-587, 2010.

Iscan, Y., Wissing, S.A., Hekimoglu, S., Müller, R.H. Solid lipid nanoparticles (SLN) for topical drug delivery: incorporation of the lipophilic drugs N,N-diethyl-m-toluamide and vitamin K. *Pharmazie,* 60: 905-909, 2005.

Jaafar-Maalej, C., Elaissari, A., Fessi, H. Lipid-based carriers: manufacturing and applications for pulmonary toute. *Expert Opin. Drug Deliv.,* 9: 1111-1127, 2012.

Jain, S., Chourasia, M.K., Masuriha, R., Soni, V., Jain, A., Jain, N.K., Gupta, Y. Solid lipid nanoparticles bearing flurbiprofen for transdermal delivery. *Drug Deliv.,* 12: 207-215, 2005.

Jain, S., Jain, S., Khare P., Gulbake, A., Bansal, D., Jain, S.K. Design and development of solid lipid nanoparticles (SLN) for topical drug delivery of an anti-fungal agent. *Drug Deliv.,* 17: 443-451, 2010.

Jee, J.P., Lim, S.J., Park, J.S., Kim, C.K. Stabilization of all-trans retinol by loading lipophilic antioxidants in solid lipid nanoparticles. *Eur. J. Pharm. Biopharm.,* 63: 134-139, 2006.

Jenning, V., Gysler, A., Schafer-Korting, M., Gohla, S.H. Vitamin A loaded solid lipid nanoparticles for topical use: occlusive properties and drug targeting to the upper skin. *Eur. J. Pharm. Biopharm.,* 49: 211-218, 2000.

Jenning, V., Gohla, S.H. Encapsulation of retinoids in solid lipid nanoparticles (SLN). *J. Microencapsul.,* 18: 149-158, 2001.

Jensen, L.B., Magnusson, E., Gunnarsson, L., Vermehren, C., Nielsen, H.M., Petersson, K. Corticosteroid solubility and lipid polarity control release from solid lipid nanoparticles. *Int. J. Pharm.,* 390: 53-60, 2010.

Jensen, L.B., Petersson, K., Nielsen, H.M. In vitro penetration properties of solid lipid nanoparticles in intact and barrier-impaired skin. *Eur. J. Pharm. Biopharm.,* 79: 68-75, 2011.

Jores, K., Mehnert, W., Dreschler, M., Bunjes, H., Johann, C., Mäder, K. Investigations on the structure of solid lipid nanoparticles (SLN) and oil-loaded solid lipid nanoparticles by photon correlation spectroscopy, field-flow fractionation and transmission electron microscopy. *J. Control. Release,* 95: 217-227, 2004.

Karavana, S.Y., Gökçe, E.H., Rençber, S., Özbal, S., Pekçetin, C., Güneri, P., Ertan, G. A new approach to the treatment of recurrent aphthous stomatitis with bioadhesive gels containing cyclosporine A solid lipid nanoparticles: in vivo/in vitro examinations.Int. J. Nanomedicine, 7:5693-5704, 2012.

Kuo, Y.C. & Wang, C.C. Cationic solid lipid nanopartciles with cholesterol-mediated surface layer for transporting saquinavir to the brain. *Biotechnol. Prog.,* 30: 198-206, 2014.

Lasa-Saracibar, B., de Mendoza, A.E.H., Guada, M., Dios-Vieitez, C., Blanco-Prieto, M.J. Lipid nanoparticles for cancer therapy: state of art and future prospects. *Expert Opin. Drug Deliv.,*9(10): 1245-1261, 2012.

Liu, J., Hu, W., Chen, H., Ni, Q., Xu, H., Yang, X. Isotretinoin-loaded solid lipid nanoparticles with skin targeting for topical delivery. *Int. J. Pharm.*, 328: 191-195, 2007.

Liu, J., Gong, T., Fu, H., Wang, C., Wang X., Chen, Q., Zhang, Q., He, Q., Zhang, Z. Solid lipid nanoparticles for pulmonary delivery of insulin. *Int. J. Pharm.*, 356: 333-344, 2008.

Lohani, A.,Verma, A., Joshi, H., Yadav, N., Kark, N. Nanotechnology-Based Cosmeceuticals.ISRN Dermatology, Volume 2014: Article ID 843687, 14 pages, 2014.

Lv, Q.,Yu, A., Xi, Y., Li, H., Song, Z., Cui, J., Cao, F., Zhai, G. Development and evaluation of penciclovir-loaded solid lipid nanoparticles fortopical delivery. *Int. J. Pharm.*, 372: 191-198, 2009.

Maia, C.S., Mehnert, W., Schafer-Korting, M. Solid lipid nanoparticles as drug carriers for topical glucocorticoids. *Int. J. Pharm.*, 196: 165-167, 2000.

Maia, C.S., Mehnert, W., Schaller, M., Korting, H.C., Gysler, A., Haberland, A., Schäfer-Korting, M. Drug targeting by solid lipid nanoparticles for dermal use. *J. Drug Target.*, 10: 489-495, 2002.

Masserini M. Nanoparticles for brain drug delivery. *ISRN Biochemistry,*Article ID 238428, 2013.

Mehnert, W. & Mader, K. Solid lipid nanoparticles: production, characterization and application. *Adv. Drug Deliv. Rev.*, 47: 165-196, 2001.

Mitri, K., Shegokar, R., Gohla, S., Anselmi, C., Müller, R.H. Lipid nanocarriers for dermal delivery of lutein: preparation, characterization, stability and performance. *Int. J. Pharm.*, 414: 267-275, 2011.

Morel, S., Terreno, E., Ugazio, E., Aime, S., Gasco, M.R. NMR relaxometric investigationsof solid lipid nanoparticles (SLN) containing gadolinium (III)complexes. *Eur. J. Pharm. Biopharm.*, 45:157–63, 1998.

Müller, R.H., Lucks, J.S. Medication vehicles made of solid lipid particles (solid lipid nanospheres-SLN). *EPO605497*, 1993.

Müller, R.H., Maaben, S., Weyhers, H., Mehnert, W. Phagocytic uptake and cytotoxicity of solid lipid nanoparticles (SLN) sterically stabilized with poloxamine 908 and poloxamer 407. *J. Drug Target.*, 4: 161-170, 1996.

Müller, R.H., Mäder, K., Gohla, S. Solid lipid nanoparticles (SLN) for controlled drug delivery-a review of the state of art. *Eur. J. Pharm. Biopharm.*,50: 161-177, 2000.

Müller, R.H., Radtke, M., Wissing, S.A. Solid lipid nanoparticles (SLN) and nanostructured lipid carriers (NLC) in cosmetic and dermatological preparations. *Adv. Drug Deliv. Rev.,* 54 (Suppl. 1): S131-S155, 2002.

Nikolic, S., Keck, C.M., Anselmi, C., Müller, R.H. Skin photoprotection improvement: synergistic interaction between lipid nanoparticles and organic UV filters. *Int. J. Pharm.,* 414: 276-284, 2011.

Padois, K., Cantieni, C., Bertholle, V., Bardel, C., Pirot, F., Falson, F. Solid lipid nanoparticles suspension versusu commercial solutions for dermal delivery of minoxidil.*Int. J. Pharm.,* 416: 300-304, 2011.

Pandey, R., Sharma, S., Khuller, G.K. Oral solid lipid nanoparticle-based antitubercular chemotherapy. *Tuberculosis,* 85(5-6): 415-420, 2005a.

Pandey, R., Khuller, G.K. Solid lipid particle-based inhalable sustained dryg delivery system against experimental tuberculosis. *Tuberculosis,* 85(4): 227-234, 2005b.

Pandita, D., Ahuja, A., Lather, V., Benjamin, B., Dutta, T., Velpandian, T., Khar, R.K. Development of lipid-based nanoparticles for enhancing the oral bioavailability of paclitaxel. *AAPS PharmSciTech*, 12: 712-722, 2011.

Passerini, N., Gavini, E., Albertini, B., Rassu, G., Di Sabatino, M., Sanna, V., Giunchedi, P., Rodriquez, L. Evaluation of solid lipid microparticles produced by spray congealing for topical application of econazole nitrate. *J. Pharm. Pharmacol.,* 61: 559-567, 2009.

Patel, S., Chavhan, S., Soni, H., Babbar, A.K., Mathur, R., Mishra, A.K., Sawant, K. Brain targeting of risperidone-loaded solid lipid nanoparticlesby intranasal route. *J. Drug Target.,* 19: 468–474, 2011.

Patil, J., Gurav, P., Kulkarni, R., Jadhav, S., Mandave, S., Shete, M., Chipade, V. Applications of solid lipid nanopraticle in novel drug delivery system. *British Biomed. Bull.,* 1: 103-118, 2013.

Pople, P.V. & Singh, K.K. Development and evaluation of tropical formulation containing solid lipid nanoparticles of Vitamin A. *AAPS PharmSciTech,* 7: E63-69, 2006.

Pople, P.V. & Singh, K.K. Targeting tacrolimus to deeper layers of skin with improved safety for treatment of atopic dermatitis. *Int. J. Pharm.,* 398: 165-178, 2010.

Puglia, C., Bonina, F., Castelli, F., Micieli, D., Sarpietro, M.G. Evaluation of percutaneous absorption of the repellent diethyltoluamide and the sunscreen ethylhexyl p-methoxycinnamate-loaded solid lipid nanoparticles: an in-vitro study. *J. Pharm. Pharmacol.,* 61: 1013-1019, 2009.

Puglia, C., Blasi, P., Rizza, L., Schoubben, A., Bonina, F., Rossi, C., Ricci, M. Lipid nanoparticles for prolonged topical delivery: an in vitro and in vivo investigation. *Int. J. Pharm.,* 357: 295-304, 2008.

Puglia, C. & Bonina, F. Lipid nanoparticles as novel delivery systems for cosmetics and dermal pharmaceuticals. *Expert Opin. Drug Deliv.,*9(4): 429-441, 2012.

Radomska-Soukharev, A. Stability of lipid excipients in solid lipid nanoparticles. *Adv. Drug Deliv. Rev.,*59: 411-418, 2007.

Ridolfi, D.M., Marcato, P.D., Machado, D., Silva, R.A., Justo, G.Z., Durán, N. In vitro cytotoxicity assays of solid lipid nanoparticles in epithelial and dermal cells. *J. Physics,*304: 012032, 2011.

Ruktanonchai, U., Bejrapha, P., Sakulkhu, U., Opanasopit, P., Bunyapraphatsara, N., Junyaprasert, V., Puttipipatkhachorn, S. Physicochemical characteristics, cytotoxicity, and antioxidant activity of three lipid nanoparticulate formulations of alpha-lipoic acid. *AAPS PharmSciTech*, 10: 227-234, 2009.

Quintanar-Guerrero, D., Tamayo-Esquivel, D., Ganem-Quintanar, A., Alléman, E., Doelker, E. Adaptation and optimization of the emulsification-diffusiontechnique to prepare lipidic nanospheres. *Eur. J. Pharm. Sci.*, 26:211–218, 2005.

Sandri, G., Bonferoni, M.C., Gökçe, E.H., Ferrari, F., Rossi, S., Patrini, M., Caramella, C. Chitosan-associated SLN: in vitro and ex vivo characterization of cyclosporine A loaded ophthalmic systems. *J. Microencapsul.,* 27: 735-746, 2010.

Sanna, V., Gavini, E., Cossu, M., Rassu, G.,Giunchedi, P. Solid lipid nanoparticles (SLN) as carriers for the topical drug delivery of econazole nitrate: in-vitro characterization, ex-vivo and in-vivo studies. *J. Pharm. Pharmacol.,*59: 1057-1064, 2007.

Schwarz, C., Mehnert, W., Lucks, J.S., Müller, R.H. Solid lipid nanoparticles (SLN) for controlled drug delivery. I. Production, characterization and sterilization. *J. Cont. Release,* 30: 83-96, 1994.

Schwarz, C. Feste lipid nanopartikel: Herstellung, charakterisierung, Arzneistoffinkorporation und –freisetzung, sterilisation und lyophilisation.Ph.D. Thesis, Free University of Berlin, 1995.

Schwarz, C. & Mehnert, W. Freeze-drying of drug-free and drug-loaded solid lipid nanoparticles (SLN). *Int. J. Pharm.,* 157: 171-179, 1997.

Schubert, M.A. & Müller-Goyman, C.C. Solvent injection as a new approach for manufacturing lipid nanopartciles – evaluation of the method and process parameters. *Eur. J. Pharm. Biopharm.,*55: 125-131, 2003.

Singh, A.P., Saraf, S.K., Saraf, A.S. SLN approach for nose to brain delivery of alprazolam. *Drug Deliv. and Transl. Res.,* 2: 498-507, 2012.

Shah, K.A., Date, A.A., Joshi, M.D., Patravale, V.B. Solid lipid nanoparticles (SLN) of tretinoin: potential in topical delivery. *Int. J. Pharm.,* 345: 163-171, 2007.

Sharma, V.K., Divan, A., Sardana, S., Dhall, V. Solid lipid nanoparticles system: an overview. *Int. J. Res. Pharm. Sci.,* 2(3): 450-461, 2011.

Sjostrom, B. & Bergenståhl, B.Preparation of submicron drug particlesin lecithin-stabilized o/w emulsions I. Model studies of the precipitationof cholesterylacetate. *Int J Pharm*, 88:53–62, 1992.

Speiser, P. Lipid nanopellets als tragersystem fur arzneimittel zur peroralen anwendung. *EPO*167825, 1990.

Souto, E.B., Wissing, S.A., Barbosa, C.M., Müller, R.H. Development of a controlled release formulation based on SLN and NLC for topical clotrimazole delivery.*Int. J. Pharm.,* 278: 71-77, 2004.

Souto, E.B., Müller, R.H., Gohla, S. A novel approach based on lipid nanoparticles (SLN) for topical delivery of alpha-lipoic acid. *J. Microencapsul.,* 22: 581-592, 2005.

Souto, E.B. & Müller, R.H. The use of SLN and NLC as topical particulte carriers for imidazole intifungal agents. *Pharmazie,* 61: 431-437, 2006.

Souto, E.B. & Müller, R.H. Rhelogical and in vitro release behaviour of clatrimazole-containing aqueous solid lipid nanoparticle dispersions and commercial creams. *Pharmazie,* 62: 505-509, 2007.

Sznitowska, M.,Janicki, S., Gajewska, M., Kulik, M. Investigation of diazepam lipospheres based on Witepsol and lecithin for oral or rectal delivery. *Acta Polon Pharm.,* 57: 61-64, 2000.

Sznitowska, M., Gajewska, M., Janicki, S., Radwanska, A., Lukowski, G. Bioavailability of diazepam from aqueous-organic solution, submicron emulsion and solid lipid nanoparticles after rectal administration in rabbits. *Eur. J. Pharm. Biopharm.,* 52: 159-163, 2001.

Trombino, S., Cassano, R., Muzzalupo, R., Pingitore, A., Cione, E., Picci, N. Stearyl ferulate-based solid lipid nanoparticles for the encapsulation and stabilization of beta –carotene and alpha –tocopherol. *Colloid Surf. B,* 72: 181-187, 2009.

Trotta, M.,Cavalli, R., Trotta, C., Bussano, R., Costa, L. Electrospray technique for solid lipid-basedparticle production. *Drug Development and Industrial Pharmacy*, 36(4): 431–438, 2010.

Uner, M., Wissing, S.A., Yener, G., Müller, R.H. Solid lipid nanoparticles (SLN) and nanostructured lipid carriers (NLC) forapplication of ascorbyl palmitate. *Pharmazie*, 60: 577-582, 2005.

Üner, M & Yener, G. Importance of solid lipid nanoparticles (SLN) in various administration routes and future perspectives. *Int. J. Nanomed.*, 2(3): 289-300, 2007.

Van Woensel, M.,Wauthoz, N., Rosière, R., Amighi, K., Mathieu, V., Lefranc, F., van Gool, S.W., de Vleeschouwer, S. Formulations for intranasal delivery of pharmacological agentsto combat brain disease: a new opportunity to tackle GBM?*Cancers*, 5: 1020-1048, 2013.

Westesen, K. & Siekmann, B. Investigation of the gel formation of phospholipid-stabilized solid lipid nanoparticles. *Int. J. Pharm.*, 151: 35-45, 1997.

Westesen, K., Bunjes, H., Koch, M.H.J. Physicochemical characterization of lipid nanoparticles and evaluation of their drug load,ng capacity and sustained release potential. *J. Control. Release*, 48: 223-236, 1997.

Westesen, K. Novel lipid-based colloidal dispersions as potential drug administration systems-expectations and reality. *Coll. Polym. Sci.*, 278: 609-618, 2000.

Wissing, S., Lippacher, A., Müller, R.H. Investigation on the occlusive properties of solid lipid nanoparticles (SLN). *J. Cosmet. Sci.*, 52: 313-324, 2001.

Wissing, S.A. & Müller, R.H. Solid lipid nanoparticles as carrier for sunscreens: in vitro release and in vivo skin penetration. *J. Control. Release*, 81: 225-233, 2002.

Wissing, S.A., Kayser, O., Müller, R.H. Solid lipid nanoparticles for parenteral drug delivery. *Adv. Drug Deliv. Rev.*, 56: 1257-1272, 2004.

Yadav, N., Khatak, S., Sara, U.V.S. Solid lipid nanaoparticles-a review. *Int. J. App. Pharm.*, 5(2): 8-18, 2013.

Yang, S.C., Lu, L.F., Cai, Y., Zhu, J.B., Liang, B.W., Yang, C.Z. Body distribution in mice of intravenously injected camptothecin solid lipid nanoparticles and targeting effect on brain. *J. Cont. Release*, 59: 299-307, 1999a.

Yang, S.C., Zhu, J., Lu, Y., Liang, B., Yang, C. Body distribution in mice of camptothecin solid lipid nanoparticles after oral administration. *Pharm. Res.,*16: 751-757, 1999b.

Zhang, J. & Smith, E. Percutaneous permeation of betamethasone 17-valerate incorporated in lipid nanopartciles. *J. Pharm. Sci.*, 100: 896-903, 2011.

Zur Mühlen A., Schwarz, C., Mehnert, W. Solid lipid nanoparticles (SLN) for controlled drug delivery-drug release and release mechanism. *Eur. J. Pharm. Biopharm.,*45: 149-155, 1998.

Zur Mühlen A. & Mehnert, W. Drug release and release mechanisms of prednisolone loaded solid lipid nanoparticles. *Pharmazie,*53: 552-555, 1998.

CHAPTER 2

DERMAL APPLICATIONS OF SOLID LIPID NANOPARTICLES (SLNs)

Ulya BADILLI

Several administration routes for SLNs have been widely investigated, including parenteral, ocular, pulmonary, oral and dermal applications. In recent years, numerous studies have been focused on the dermal application of SLNs for pharmaceutical and cosmetic purposes due to their unique features and advantages. This chapter provides an overview of dermal application of SLNs inboth pharmaceutic and cosmetic fields.

Dermal Applications of SLNs in Pharmaceutics

Topical application of drugs for skin diseases offers some advantages, such as achieving high drug levels at the target site and reducingsystemic side effects. However, the physicochemical properties of the drug and the vehicle are the primary limiting factors for percutaneous absorption and penetration of the drug. Nano-sized drug delivery systems, including lipid nanoparticles, are receiving increasing attention as a way to overcome these limitations and to provide efficient and site-specific skin targeting.

SLNs have numerous advantages for dermal application. They can provide controlled release profiles for many drugs. They have an excellent tolerability because they are composed of physiological and biodegradable lipids. They can enhance percutaneous absorption and provide efficient drug targetingto the different skin layers (Pardeike et al., 2009). Application of an SLN dispersion to the skin surface results in formation of an occlusive film layer on the skin due to the evaporation of water from the nanodispersion. This occlusive feature of the SLNs is a function of the small size and strong adhesive properties of the particles. The occlusive film formed on the skin reduces transepidermal water loss and increases the hydration of the stratum corneum layer, thereby facilitating the penetration of drugs into deeper skin strata. The small size also ensures a close contact with the stratum corneum and consequently enhances the amount of drug penetrated into the skin (Schafer-Korting et al., 2007; Gupta et al., 2012). Lipid nanoparticles can also enhance the chemical stability of active substances that are sensitive to light, oxidation or hydrolysis (Müller et al., 2000).

Commonly Used Dermal Active Ingredients in SLNs

Topical Corticosteroids

Glucocorticoids are widely used for the treatment of several skin diseases, such as atopic dermatitis, eczema and psoriasis. Santos Maia et al. (2002) investigated SLNs as a drug delivery system for topical application of a glucocorticoid, prednicarbate. They demonstrated that prednicarbate targeting to the viable epidermis could be achieved by SLNs. They also expressed that a better benefit/risk ratio could be expected for the topical application of prednicarbate loaded SLN because the inflammatory process is most pronounced within the epidermis and the glucocorticoid located in the dermis is responsible for the induction of irreversible skin atrophy.

Bikkad et al. (2014) loaded halobetasol propionate, a high potency synthetic topical corticosteroid, into a SLN formulation by solvent injection method. These SLNs were successfully incorporated into the polymeric Carbopol® gels for topical application. The SLN based topical gel exhibited low skin irritation, high occlusivity and controlled drug release when compared with Carbopol ®974 P gel as well as a market product.

Jensen et al. (2011) prepared betamethasone-17-valerate loaded SLN formulations and evaluated them using intact and barrier-impaired porcine skin. The amount of betamethasone retained in the intact and barrier-impaired skin was increased and a reservoir of the drug in the stratum corneum layer was created with the SLN formulation. High levels of betamethasone in the skin were achieved by administration of the SLN formulation when compared with an ointment.

Antifungal Agents

Antifungal agents are one of the most effective active ingredient groups applied by the dermal route. Among these are undecylenic acid and copper salts, benzoic acid and salicylic acid, phenolic compounds, imidazole derivative compounds, nystatin and candicidin (Barry, 1983).

Terbinafine is an antifungal agent with a potent broad-spectrum fungicidal activity arising from inhibition of squalene epoxidase. Terbinafine-loaded SLNs were formulated using different solid lipids. The application of this SLN formulation prepared with a 4% lipid phase containing a mixture of glyceryl monostearate and Compritol[®] 888 (1:1) for 12 hours showed a comparable efficacy to that of LamisilOnce[®] application for 24 hours, which would resolve the practical problem of the longer administration period required with LamisilOnce[®] (Chen et al., 2012).

Wavikar and Vavia (2013) also prepared and evaluated a SLN-based topical nanolipid gel containing terbinafine hydrochloride. The researchers reported that the SLN-based nanolipid gel provides an increased skin deposition, improves in vitro antimicotic activity. The prepared gel also facilitates impressive occlusion properties without skin irritation.

Miconazole nitrate is one of the broad-spectrum antifungal agents typically applied for the topical treatment of dermatophytoses and superficial mycoses. A hydrogel bearing miconazole nitrate-loaded SLNs was developed by Jain et al. (2010) for topical application. This SLN-bearing hydrogel formulation provided sustained release of miconazole nitrate. In addition, greater drug deposition into the skin and better in vivo antifungal efficiency with less erythemal score were achieved with topical administration of the SLN formulation.

Sanna et al. (2007) designed SLN formulations of econazole nitrate for topical administration. The results ofin vivostudies confirmed that SLN promoted a rapid penetration of econazole nitrate through the stratum corneum after one hour and improved the diffusion of the drug in the deeper skin layers after three hours, when compared with the reference gel formulation. These SLNs were considered useful for site-specific delivery of drugs to the skin.

Vitamin A Derivatives

Vitamin A and its derivatives are widely used and important compounds for treatment of various skin conditions, such as psoriasis, skin cancer and photoaging. These compounds play an important role in the treatment of skin diseases due to their antioxidant properties and other mechanisms of action (Keller et al., 1998).

Jenning et al. (2000) evaluated the potential use of retinol-loaded SLNs in dermatology. SLNs were incorporated into a hydrogel and o/w cream and tested for their drug penetration efficacy. Application of SLN formulations resulted in high drug concentrations in the upper skin layers whereas very low retinol levels were present in the lower skin layers.

Shah et al. (2007) tested tretinoin-loaded SLN formulations for skin irritation in rabbits and found that SLN based tretinoin gel was significantly less irritating to skin. The researchers claimed that the skin tolerability of tretinoin could be improved by the use of SLN formulations.

Anti-inflammatory Drugs

Nonsteroidal anti-inflammatory drugs are the most commonly used agents for treatment of rheumatic diseases and other inflammation-caused conditions. Since most skin diseases are caused by inflammation, these agents have an important place in dermatology practice (Friedman et al., 2002).

Meloxicam is a potent non-steroidal anti-inflammatory drug and its dermal application is a preferred option for reducing the gastrointestinal and systemic side effects of drug. Khurana et al. (2013) investigated SLNs as a way to obtain an effective dermal delivery of meloxicam. They demonstrated that the SLN-gel formulation of meloxicam showed notable anti-inflammatory activity and perfect skin tolerability. They concluded that SLNs could be preferred for the dermal delivery of non-steroidal anti-inflammatory drugs to prevent systemic side effects.

Another study that used meloxicam-loaded SLN formulations examined the effects of lipid type and concentration and the surfactant ratios on the physicochemical properties of SLNs and their active ingredient release profiles. The SLNs were prepared using modified high-shear homogenisation and ultrasonication methods. Either Geleol, Compritol 888 ATO or Precirol ATO5 were used as the lipid in these formulations and Poloxamer 188 was the surfactant. The meloxicam-loaded SLNs had an active compound-enriched core and a particle size that varied between 325-1080 nm. In vitro dissolution studies showed that meloxicam was continuously released from the SLNs for up to 48 hours. These SLNs were concluded to have excellent physical stabilities and high encapsulation effectiveness for topical application of meloxicam and they were regarded as promising carrier systems for controlled active ingredient release (Khalil et al., 2013).

Jain et al. (2005) prepared flurbiprofen-loaded SLNs for transdermal delivery to manage the inflammation and pain of osteoarthritis and rheumatoid arthritis. An SLN dispersion and an SLN-based gel formulation of flurbiprofen displayed sustained drug release over 24 hours; however, this effect was greater for the gel formulation. The percent inhibition of oedema after 8 hours was significantly higher with the gel formulation than for flurbiprofen alone or the SLN dispersion of the drug. The SLN based gel formulation significantly decreased the inflammation and also sustained this effect.

Miscellaneous

The frequently used active ingredients mentioned above are the basic substances for dermal applications. Other dermal SLN application studies have been conducted with different active ingredients. For example, podophyllotoxin is the first-line drug for the treatment of genital warts since it can inhibit the growth of epithelial cell infected by human papilloma virus in epidermis. Chen et al. (2006) compared a podophyllotoxin-loaded SLN formulation with a podophyllotoxin tincture for their epidermal targeting effects. They found that podophyllotoxin was located in the epidermis and no drug was observed in the dermis after SLN application. The localisation of the drug in the epidermis and a reduction in the systemic side effects with SLN formulation were suggested by these researchers.

Tacrolimus is an effective macrolide immunosuppressant for the immune-inflammatory diseases. Pople and Singh (2010) prepared and evaluated lipid nanoparticles containing tacrolimus. The authors reporteda significantly enhanced penetration to the deeper skin layers and accumulation of an effective amount of drug at the target site for atopic dermatitis following application of an SLN formulation. In addition, no skin irritation was observed and improved safety was obtained with lipid nanoparticles of tacrolimus.

Minoxidil is a pyridine derivative commonly used for the topical treatment of androgenic alopecia. Padois et al. (2011) investigated the potential of SLNs as a drug delivery system for minoxidil and found the SLN dispersions of minoxidil to be as efficient as the tested commercial products. The SLN formulations, unlike the commercial products, were also completely non-irritant because they were prepared using physiological lipids and solvent-free techniques.

Penciclovir, a synthetic nucleoside analogue, is a potent and highly selective inhibitor of herpes viruses such as herpes simplex virus, Epstein-Barr virus and cytomegalovirus. Lv et al. (2009) studied the skin targeting behaviours of penciclovir-loaded SLN formulations. The amount of penciclovir penetrated into the dermis from SLNs at 12 h was 2.3 fold higher than that achieved with a commercial cream product.

Table 1. List of research related to solid lipid nanoparticles for topical drug delivery.

Lipid	Drug	Indication	Findings	Reference
Precirol ATO, cetyl palmitate, Dynasan 116	Betamethasone-17-valerate	Atopic dermatitis	The amount of betamethasone retained in the intact and barrier-impaired skin could be increased and a reservoir of the drug in the stratum corneum layer could be created with SLN.	Jensen et al. (2011)
Monostearin, Beeswax	Betamethasone-17-valerate	Inflammatory skin diseases	Corticosteroid could be targeted specifically to the inflammatory site in the upper layers of the skin with monostearin SLN.	Zhang and Smith (2011)
Glyceryl monostearate	Halobetasol propionate	Psoriasis	SLN based topical gel exhibited low skin irritation, high occlusivity and controlled drug release as compared with a conventional gel and market product.	Bikkad et al. (2014)
Compritol 888 ATO, Precirol, Witepsol, Dynasan 114	Prednicarbate	Atopic dermatitis	Prednicarbate targeting to the viable epidermis and better benefit/risk ratio were obtained with the topical application of prednicarbate loaded SLN.	Santos Maia et al. (2002)
Dynasan 114	Tacrolimus	Atopic dermatitis	Enhanced penetration into the deeper skin layers and effective amounts of the drug in the target site was obtained with lipid nanoparticles.	Pople and Singh (2010)
Compritol 888 ATO	Fluconazole	Cutaneous candidiasis	SLNs containing fluconazole showed better antifungal activity in consequence of the localised drug-depot formation in skin and controlled release of the drug.	Gupta et al. (2013)
Compritol 888 ATO, Precirol ATO 5, Glyceryl	Miconazole nitrate	Fungal infection	The gel formulation containing miconazole loaded SLN provided higher amounts of	Bhalekar et al. (2009)

monostearate			drug localised in the skin in comparison with a conventional gel.	
Tristearin	Miconazole nitrate	Fungal infection	Higher drug deposition into skin and better *in vivo* antifungal efficiency with less erythemal score were achieved with the SLN formulation.	Jain et al. (2010)
Precirol ATO 5	Econazole nitrate	Fungal infection	SLN enhanced the penetration of drug through the stratum corneum after 1hour and improved the diffusion in the deeper skin layers after 3 hours.	Sanna et al. (2007)
Dynasan 116	Clotrimazole	Model drug	SLN showed a superior occlusive capacity and it could be also used for modified release of lipophilic drugs.	Souto et al. (2004)
Compritol 888 ATO, glyceryl monostearate, Precirol ATO 5	Terbinafine	Tinea pedis (Athlete's foot)	Application of SLN containing the mixture of glyceryl monostearate and Compritol 888 for 12 hours had a comparable efficiency with LamisilOnce® for 24 hours. The practical problem of the longer administration period necessary for the commercial product could be resolved.	Chen et al. (2012)
Glyceryl monostearate	Terbinafine hydrochloride	Superficial fungal infection	Enhanced skin deposition, improved *in vitro* antimicotic activity and effective occlusion properties obtained with SLN-based gel formulation.	Wavikar, Vavia (2013)
Compritol 888 ATO	All-trans retinoic acid	Acne	Retinoic acid loaded SLN enabled comedolytic effects and decreased retinoic acid-induced skin irritation without reducing the efficacy of drug.	Castro et al. (2011)
Precirol ATO 5	Isotretinoin	Acne	SLN formulation of isotretinoin containing 3% Precirol ATO, 4% soybean lecithin and 4.5% Tween 80 significantly increased the accumulative amount of the drug in the skin and	Liu et al. (2007)

			demonstrated an improved skin-targeting effect.	
Glyceryl monostearate, Compritol 888 ATO, Dynasan 116	Tretinoin	Inflammatory skin diseases	Skin tolerability and photostability of tretinoin could be dramatically improved with SLN.	Shah et al. (2007)
Compritol 888 ATO	Retinol	Model drug	High drug concentrations in the upper skin layers were obtained while very low retinol levels were present in the lower skin layers with SLN.	Jenning et al. (2000)
Cetyl palmitate	Meloxicam	Arthritis	SLN based gel formulation containing meloxicam showed an important anti-inflammatory activity and great skin tolerability.	Khurana et al. (2013)
Stearic acid, cholesterol	Flurbiprofen	Osteoarthritis, rheumatoid arthritis	The percent inhibition of oedema after 8 hours was significantly higher with an SLN-based gel when compared with flurbiprofen or SLN dispersion of the drug.	Jain et al. (2005)
Cetyl palmitate	Idebenone	Skin oxidative damages	Idebenone-loaded SLNs could target the drug to the upper skin layers and improve the bioavailability after topical application.	Montenegro et al. (2012)
Tripalmitin	Podophyllotoxin	Genital warts	Podophyllotoxin was located in the epidermis and no drug was observed in the dermis after SLN application. As a result, reduction in the systemic side effects with SLN formulation was suggested.	Chen et al. (2006)
Semi-synthetic triglycerides (Suppocire® NAI50)	Minoxidil	Androgenic alopecia	SLN formulations were completely non-corrosive when compared with commercial products.	Padois et al. (2011)
Glyceryl monostearate	Penciclovir	Herpes simplex virus infection	The amount of penciclovir penetrated into dermis from SLNs was 2.3 fold greater compared with commercial	Lv et al. (2009)

				cream.	
Compritol 888 ATO, ATO 5	Precirol	Lidocaine	Local anaesthetic effect	Lipid nanoparticles significantly sustained the drug release compared to commercial gel product. A gel formulation containing lidocaine-loaded SLNs provided a five-fold increase in duration of anaesthesia when compared with a commercial gel.	Pathak and Nagarsenker (2009)
Tristearin glyceride, stearic acid		Triptolide	Inflammatory and autoimmune diseases	The anti-inflammatory effect of triptolide in SLN-hydrogel was over two-fold higher than that of a conventional hydrogel of the drug.	Mei et al. (2005)

Cosmetic Applications of SLNs

SLNs have been introduced as potent carrier systems not only for various drugs but also for cosmetic active ingredients. SLNs are promising carriers for cosmetics and cosmeceuticals because they have a number of superior properties when compared withconventional formulations. For example, they are capable of protecting the unstable cosmetic compounds from degradation. Controlled release of cosmeceuticals is also possible with SLNs depending on the SLN type (e.g. SLNs with drug-enriched shells or drug-enriched cores). A burst release could be obtained with the drug-enriched shell type of SLNs whereas the drug-enriched core types of SLNs would lead to sustained release.

SLNs have obvious occlusive properties because of the formation of a perfect film as the formulations dry, and this characteristic depends on the particle size, lipid crystallisation and lipid concentration of the SLNs. Consequently, SLNs can be used to enhance the water content of the skin. The occlusive effect also stimulates the penetration of cosmetic active ingredients into the upper layer of the epidermis, especially the stratum corneum. SLNs can also act as physical sunscreens on their own because they have a UV-blocking potential. They can also be used for the encapsulation of molecular sunscreens, thereby improving the photoprotective effect of the sunscreen (Wissing and Müller, 2003a).

Occlusion and skin hydration effects of SLNs

Submicron sized particles form a monolayer film when they are appliedto theskin because of their adhesive properties. This film layer has an occlusive effect on the skin that is dependent on the SLN particle size. Comparison of a layer of nanoparticles compared with a layer of microparticles reveals that the nanoparticles have air channels with much smaller dimensions. This will decrease the evaporation of water, thereby increasing skin hydration (Souto and Müller, 2008). Wissing et al. (2001) demonstrated that various factors, such as particle size, applied sample volume (lipid mass), lipid concentration and crystallinity of the lipid,play important roles in the occlusive effect of SLNs. They introduced optimum conditions of a particle size of 200 nm, a minimum lipid mass of 3.7 mg/cm^2 and high degree of crystallinity of the lipid that provided optimum occlusive properties.

The influence of SLNs on skin hydration and viscoelasticity was evaluated by Wissing and Müller (2003b). An O/W cream containing SLN and a conventional O/W cream were compared in terms of their improvement of skin hydration and viscoelasticity. These in vivo studies showed that the cream formulation enriched with SLNs significantly increased the skin hydration when compared with the conventional cream after 4 weeks of treatment.

SLNs as carrier systems for cosmetic active agents

Prolonged release of perfumes and fragrance materials offers the advantage for once-a-day application and could be made possible with SLNs. Wissing et al. (2000) encapsulated the perfume Allure (Chanel) in SLNs and demonstrated a prolonged release of perfume from the lipid nanoparticles when compared with the oil droplets of an emulsion. After 6 hours, the perfume was completely released from the emulsion formulation while only 75% of the perfume was released from SLNs in the same period.

Topical use of caffeine, a natural alkaloid found in tea leaves, coffee, cocoa and kola nuts, has attracted great attention in cosmetics for anti-cellulite purposes. However, caffeine, because of its hydrophilic character, does not readily penetrate through the stratum corneum. Puglia et al. (2014) evaluated SLNs as a carrier system for topical application of caffeine. They concluded that a significantly faster permeation occurred with caffeine loaded SLNs than with a reference gel. The caffeine amount delivered to the receptor phase over 24 h was significantly greater with SLNsthan with the gel formulation.

Dingler et al. (1999) revealed that the penetration of vitamin E into the skin was improved by means of the occlusion effect of SLN. The chemical stability of vitamin E was also increased with lipid nanoparticles. The SLNs also showed an excellent pigment effect and concealed the undesired brown colour of vitamin E.

Alpha-lipoic acid is a natural substance that inhibits cross-linking between proteins and other large molecules responsible for the ageing process. It is also less irritating than other anti-aging actives like hydroxy acids, so skin care products containing alpha-lipoic acid are drawing great interest. However, lipoic acid is chemically unstable and its degradation products are responsible for an unpleasant odour in cosmetics. Souto et al. (2005a) evaluated the use of SLNs for encapsulation of lipoic acid in cosmetic formulations by characterising the particle size and thermal and rheological properties and conducting UV measurements.

Coenzyme Q10 is a lipophilic endogenous antioxidant. Its low aqueous solubility and the barrier function of the stratum corneum complicate the preparation of a formulation that is able to delivercoenzyme Q10 to deeper layers of the skin. Korkmaz et al. (2013) prepared SLN formulations containing coenzyme Q10 using a high speed homogenisation method and incorporated the SLNs into Carbopol 974P hydrogels. Trolox equivalent antioxidant capacity (TEAC) analysis confirmed that the antioxidant performance of coenzyme Q10 could be preserved in SLNs. Rheological characterisation demonstrated that gel formulations including SLN were shear thinning and suitable for topical application in terms of their mechanical strength. The amount of coenzyme Q10 absorbed by the skin was increased two-fold with an SLN-based gel formulation when compared to the gel containing pure active agent. The SLNs were concluded to be successful carriers for delivering coenzyme Q10 efficiently into the skin without loss of antioxidant activity.

Farboud et al. (2011) compared the use of a conventional cream formulation of coenzyme Q10 with a cream containing coenzyme Q10-loaded SLNs on volunteers. In vitro release studies showed that prolonged release of this substance was achieved with SLNs. Higher increases in skin humidity and elasticity, which are desirable effects for anti-wrinkle products, were obtained with a cream formulation consisting of SLNs.

Protection from the harmful effects of UV radiation is important point for human health. Sunscreens should act on the surface of the skin and show insignificant penetration to the deeper skin layers. The extent of penetration depends not only on the physicochemical properties of the sunscreen but also on the properties of the carrier system. One of the most important fields of applications of SLNs is their usage in sunscreen formulations. SLNs act as physical sunscreens on their own and provide a synergistic effect on UV protection when they are used for encapsulation of the molecular sunscreens. Wissing and Müller (2002) developed oxybenzone-loaded SLN formulations and evaluated the release profile and percutaneous absorption of the sunscreen. The release rate was decreased by 30–60% with SLN formulations when compared to the conventional O/W emulsions. The amount of oxybenzone penetrated into human skin was higher from the emulsion formulations. SLN formulations formed a film layer on the skin surface and fixed the oxybenzone molecules within the film layer.

In other research, tocopherol acetate, as a chemical sunscreen, was encapsulated in SLNs to preventchemical degradation and to enhance the UV blocking capacity. Placebo SLN dispersions showed greater UV blocking effects than did tocopherol acetate-loaded emulsions. On the other hand, tocopherol acetate-loaded SLN formulations provided a synergistic additive effect (Wissing and Müller, 2001).

Carlotti et al. (2005) prepared octyl methoxycinnamate-loaded SLNs for enhancing the photostability of the sunscreen. The rate of photodegradation was determined spectrophotometrically. Protection of the molecular sunscreen against photodegradation induced by UVB radiation was achieved with SLNs.

Lacatusu et al. (2010) produced SLN formulations loaded with various UVA and UVB filters. They concluded that the encapsulation of 2-ethylhexyl trans-4-methoxycinnamate (OMC), 2-ethylhexyl-2-cyano-3,3-diphenylacrylate (OCT) and Bis-ethylhexyloxyphenol methoxyphenyl triazine (BEMT) into SLNs provided an extra additive efficiency tothese sunscreens.

Ferulic acid can be used as a UV blocking agent in anti-aging cosmetic products. It is an attractive novel sunscreen molecule, but it cannot be encapsulated into SLNs because of its oil-insoluble nature. Therefore, a lipidic ester of ferulic acid, n-dodecyl-ferulate, was synthesised by Souto et al. (2005b). SLNs containing n-dodecyl-ferulate were successfully prepared and a physical stability of at least three weeks was demonstrated for the aqueous SLN dispersion.

Cengiz et al. (2006) prepared SLN and hybrid SLN formulations containing titanium dioxide (TiO_2), which is an inert and inorganic UV filter. The SLNs were evaluated for stability and for their physicochemical characteristics. UV protection efficiencies were determined with Transpore[TM] and Sun To See[TM] techniques. All

SLN formulations showed higher UV protection effects than emulsion formulations, but the best results were obtained with hybrid SLN formulations. Stable, safe and highly efficient sunscreen formulations could be produced by the encapsulation of TiO_2 in SLNs.

REFERENCES

Barry, B.W. Dermatological Formulations. Percutaneous Absorption. Marcel Dekker Inc., New York, Chapter 1, 1983.

Bhalekar, M.R., Pokharkar, V., Madgulkar, A., Patil, N., Patil, N. Preparation and evaluation of miconazole nitrate loaded solid lipid nanoparticles for topical delivery. *AAPS PharmSciTech*, 10(1): 289 - 296, 2009.

Bikkad, M.L., Nathani, A.H., Mandlik, S.K., Shrotriya, S.N., Ranpise, N.S. Halobetasol propionate loaded solid lipid nanoparticles (SLN) for skin targeting by topical delivery. *J. Liposome Res.*, 24(2): 113-123, 2014.

Carlotti, M.E., Sapino, S., Vione, D., Pelizzetti, E., Ugazio, E., Morel, S. Study on the photostability of octyl-p-methoxy cinnamate in SLN. *Journal of Dispersion Science and Technology*, 26: 809-816, 2005.

Castro, G.A., Oliveira, C.A., Mahecha, G.A.B., Ferreira, L.A.M. Comedolytic effect and reduced skin irritation of a new formulation of all-trans retinoic acid loaded solid lipid nanoparticles for topical treatment of acne. *Arch. Dermatol. Res.*, 303: 513-520, 2011.

Cengiz, E., Wissing, S.A., Müller, R.H., Yazan, Y. Sunblocking efficiency of various TiO2 loaded solid lipid nanoparticle formulations. *Int. J. Cosmet. Sci.*, 28: 371-378, 2006.

Chen, H., Chang, X., Du, D., Liu, W., Liu, J., Weng, T., Yang, Y., Xu, H., Yang, X. Podophyllotoxin loaded solid lipid nanoparticles for epidermal targeting. *J. Control. Release*, 110: 296-306, 2006.

Chen, Y-C., Liu, D-Z., Liu, J-J., Chang, T-W., Ho, H-O., Sheu, M-T. Development of terbinafine solid lipid nanoparticles as a topical delivery system. *International Journal of Nanomedicine*, 7: 4409-4418, 2012.

Dingler, A., Blum, R.P., Niehus, H., Müller, R.H., Gohla, S. Solid lipid nanoparticles (SLN^{TM} / $Lipopearls^{TM}$) – a pharmaceutical and cosmetic carrier for the application of vitamin E in dermal products. *J. Microencapsul.*, 16(6): 751-767, 1999.

Farboud, E.S., Nasrollahi, S.A., Tabbakhi, Z. Novel formulation and evaluation of a Q10 loaded solid lipid nanoparticle cream: in vitro and in vivo studies. *Int. J. Nanomed.,* 6: 611-617, 2011.

Firedman, E.S., LaNatra, N., Stiller, M.J. NSAIDs in dermatologic therapy: review nd preview. *J. Cutan. Med. Surg.,* 6: 449-459, 2002.

Gupta, M., Agrawal, U., Vyas, S.P. Nanocarrier based topical drug delivery for the treatment of skin diseases. *Expert Opin. Drug Deliv.,* 9(7): 783-804, 2012.

Gupta, M., Tiwari, S., Vyas, S.P. Influence of various lipid core on characteristics of SLNs designed for topical delivery of fluconazole against cutaneous candidiasis, *Pharm. Dev. Tech.,* 18(3): 550-559, 2013.

Jain, S.K., Chourasia, M.K., Masuriha, R., Soni, V., Jain, A., Jain, N.K., Gupta, Y. Solid lipid nanoparticle bearing flurbiprofen for transdermal delivery. *Drug Delivery,* 12: 207-215, 2005.

Jain, S., Jain, S., Khare, P., Gulbake, A., Bansal, D., Jain, S.K. Design and development of solid lipid nanoparticles for topical delivery of an antifungal agent. *Drug Delivery,* 17(6): 443-451, 2010.

Jenning, V., Gysler, A., Schäfer-Korting, M., Gohla, S.H. Vitamin A loaded solid lipid nanoparticles for topical use: occlusive properties and drug targeting to the upper skin. *Eur. J. Pharm. Biopharm.,* 49: 211-218, 2000.

Jensen, L.B., Petersson, K., Nielsen, H.M. In vitro penetration properties of solid lipid nanoparticles in intact and barrier-impaired skin. *Eur. J. Pharm. Biopharm.,* 79: 68-75, 2011.

Keller, K.L., Fenske, N.A. Uses of vitamins A, C, and E and related compounds in dermatology: A review. *Journal of American Academy of Dermatology,* 39: 611-625, 1998.

Khalil, R.M., Abd El-Bary, A., Kassem, M.A., Ghorab, M.M. Ahmed, M.B. Solid lipid nanoparticles for topical delivery of meloxicam: development and in vitro characterization. 1st Annual International Interdisciplinary Conference, AIIC24-26 April, Azores, Portugal – Proceedings, 779-798, 2013.

Khurana, S., Bedi, P.M.S., Jain, N.K. Preparation and evaluation of solid lipid nanoparticles based nanogel for dermal delivery of meloxicam. *Chemistry and Physics of Lipids,* 175-176: 65-72, 2013.

Korkmaz, E., Gökçe, E.H., Özer, Ö. Development and evaluation of coenzyme Q10 loaded solid lipid nanoparticle hydrogel for enhanced dermal delivery. *Acta Pharm.,* 63: 517-529, 2013.

Lacatusu, I., Badea, N., Murariu, A., Bojin, D., Meghea, A. Effect of UV sunscreens loaded in solid lipid nanoparticles: a combined SPF assay and photostability. *Mol. Cryst. Liq. Cryst.*, 523: 247-259, 2010.

Liu, J., Hu, W., Chen, H., Ni, Q., Xu, H., Yang, X. Isotretinoin loaded solid lipid nanoparticles with skin targeting for topical delivery. *Int. J. Pharm.*, 328: 191-195, 2007.

Lv, Q., Yu, A., Xi, Y., Li, H., Song, Z., Cui, J., Cao, F., Zhai, G. Development and evaluation of penciclovir loaded solid lipid nanoparticles for topical delivery. *Int. J. Pharm.*, 372: 191-198, 2009.

Mei, Z., Wu, Q., Hu, S., Li, X. Triptolide loaded solid lipid nanoparticle hydrogel for topical application. *Drug Dev. Ind. Pharm.*, 31: 161-168, 2005.

Müller, R.H., Mäder, K., Gohla, S. Solid lipid nanoparticles (SLN) for controlled drug delivery-a review of the state of art. *Eur. J. Pharm. Biopharm.*, 50: 161-177, 2000.

Montenegro, L., Sinico, C., Castangia, I., Carbone, C., Puglisi, G. Idebenone loaded solid lipid nanoparticles for drug delivery to the skin: in vitro evaluation. *Int. J. Pharm.*, 434: 169-174, 2012.

Padois, K., Cantieni, C., Bertholle, V., Bardel, C., Pirot, F., Falson, F. Solid lipid nanoparticles suspension versus commercial solutions for dermal delivery of minoxidil. *Int. J. Pharm.*, 416: 300-304, 2011.

Pardeike, J., Hommoss, A., Müller, R.H. Lipid nanoparticles (SLN, NLC) in cosmetic and pharmaceutical dermal products. *Int. J. Pharm.*, 366: 170-184, 2009.

Pathak, P., Nagarsenker, M. Formulation and evaluation of lidocaine lipid nanosystems for dermal delivery. *AAPS PharmSciTech*, 10(3): 985-992, 2009.

Pople, P.V., Singh, K.K. Targeting tacrolimus to deeper layers of skin with improved safety for treatment of atopic dermatitis. *Int. J. Pharm.*, 398: 165-178, 2010.

Puglia, C., Bonina, F. Lipid nanoparticles as novel delivery systems for cosmetics and dermal pharmaceuticals. *Expert Opin. Drug Deliv.*, 9(4): 429-441, 2012.

Puglia, C., Offerta, A., Tirendi, G.G., Tarico, M.S., Curreri, S., Bonina, F., Perrotta, R.E. Design of solid lipid nanoparticles for caffeine topical administration. *Drug Delivery*, DOI: 10.3109/10717544.2014.903011.

Sanna, V., Gavini, E., Cossu, M., Rassu, G., Giunchedi, P. Solid lipid nanoparticles (SLN) as carriers for the topical delivery of econazole nitrate: in vitro characterization, ex vivo and in vivo studies. *J. Pharm. Pharmacol.*, 59: 1057-1064, 2007.

Santos Maia, C., Mehnert, W., Schaller, M., Korting, H.C., Gysler, A., Haberland, A., Schäfer-Korting, M. Drug targeting by solid lipid nanoparticles for dermal use. *Journal of Drug Targeting,* 10(6): 489-495, 2002.

Schäfer-Korting, M., Mehnert, W.,Korting, H.C. Lipid nanoparticles for improved topical application of drugs for skin diseases. *Adv. Drug Del. Rev.,* 59: 427-443, 2007.

Shah, K.A., Date, A.A., Joshi, M.D., Patravale, V.B. Solid lipid nanoparticles (SLN) of tretinoin: potential in topical delivery. *Int. J. Pharm.,* 345: 163-171, 2007.

Souto, E.B., Wissing, S.A., Barbosa, C.M., Müller, R.H. Development of a controlled release formulation based on SLN and NLC for topical clotrimazole delivery. *Int. J. Pharm.,* 278: 71-77, 2004.

Souto, E.B., Müller, R.H., Gohla, S. A novel approach based on lipid nanoparticles (SLN) for topical delivery of α-lipoic acid. *J. Microencapsul.,* 22(6): 581-592, 2005a.

Souto, E.B., Anselmi, C., Centini, M., Müller, R.H. Preparation and characterization of n-dodecyl-ferulate loaded solid lipid nanoparticles (SLN*). Int. J. Pharm.,* 295: 261-268, 2005b.

Souto, E.B., Müller, R.H. Cosmetic features and applications of lipid nanoparticles (SLN, NLC). *Int. J. Cosmet. Sci.,* 30: 157-165, 2008.

Wavikar, P., Vavia, P. Nanolipidgel for enhanced skin deposition and improved antifungal activity. *AAPS PharmSciTech,* 14(1): 222-233, 2013.

Wissing, S.A., Mäder, K., Müller, R.H. Solid lipid nanoparticles (SLN^{TM}) as a novel carrier system offering prolonged release of the perfume Allure (Chanel). *Proc. Int. Symp. Control. Rel. Bioact. Mater.,* 27: 311-312, 2000.

Wissing, S.A., Lippacher, A., Müller, R.H. Investigations on the occlusive properties of solid lipid nanoparticles (SLN). *J. Cosmet. Sci.,* 52: 313-324, 2001.

Wissing, S.A., Müller, R.H. A novel sunscreen system based on tocopherol acetate incorporated into solid lipid nanoparticles. *Int. J. Cosmet. Sci.,* 23: 233-243, 2001.

Wissing, S.A., Müller, R.H. Solid lipid nanoparticles as carrier for sunscreens: in vitro release and in vivo skin penetration. *J. Control. Release,* 81: 225-233, 2002.

Wissing, S.A., Müller, R.H. Cosmetic applications for solid lipid nanoparticles (SLN). *Int. J. Pharm.,* 254: 65-68, 2003a.

Wissing, S.A., Müller, R.H. The influence of solid lipid nanoparticles on skin hydration and viscoelasticity – in vivo study. *Eur. J. Pharm. Biopharm.,* 56: 67-72, 2003b.

Zhang, J., Smith, E. Percutaneous permeation of betamethasone-17-valerate incorporated in lipid nanoparticles. *J. Pharm. Sci.*, 100(3): 896-903, 2011.

CHAPTER 3

NOVEL DOSAGE FORMS: SEMISOLID SLNs

Ulya BADILLI, Ceyda Tuba SENGEL-TURK, Nilufer TARIMCI

As mentioned in Chapter 2, the dermal route is commonly used for local and systemic delivery of various drugs. Several recent studies have focused on topical applications of SLNs for local or systemic effects (Schäfer-Korting et al., 2007; Souto et al., 2007; Prow et al, 2011). However, SLN dispersions should be incorporated into conventional dosage forms to provide dosages with the desired semisolid consistency for topical applications. Thus, various studies have investigated the preparation of semisolid topical formulations by addition of drug-loaded SLN dispersions into cream or hydrogel vehicles. Dingler et al. (1999) produced Vitamin E loaded SLN formulations by a high pressure homogenisation technique and incorporated the SLN dispersion into a dermal O/W cream. They reported that the chemical stability of Vitamin E was significantly improved when Vitamin E was encapsulated in SLNs. According to the in vitro occlusion test data, the occlusion factor for the plain O/W cream at the 48th hour of approximately 20. Addition of the Vitamin E loaded SLNs to the O/W cream yields a distinctly high occlusion effect with an occlusion factor of about 50, which in turn increased the penetration of the active ingredient through the stratum corneum. Consequently, the researchers concluded that topical cream formulations of Vitamin E-loaded SLNs had significant advantages compared to conventional dosage forms (Dingler et al., 1999).

Another research group (Jenning et al., 2000) prepared both hydrogel and O/W cream formulations containing Vitamin A-encapsulated SLNs as new topical dosage forms. In this study, 10% glycerol, 20% SLN dispersion, 0.5% xanthan gum and water were used to fabricate the hydrogel. However, significant changes were observed in the particle size of the SLNs because of the interactions occurring between the SLN formulations and the xantham gum as a gel-forming polymer. On the other hand, particle size measurements in O/W cream formulation were more difficult to carry out and a bimodal size distribution was observed due to the presence of oil droplets.

Similar studies also have been realised by several researchers; for example, Santos Maia et al., (2002) prepared prednicarbate -a topical glucocorticoid- loaded SLNs and incorporated this system into the O/W cream formulation. These researchers concluded that SLNs are appropriate carrier systems for targeting prednicarbate to live epidermis. Mei et al. (2005) formulated a hydrogel formulation includingSLNs containing the anti-inflammatory drugtriptolide. The 12th hour cumulative transdermal absorption rate of hydrogels prepared with triptolide-loaded SLNs was 73.5%, whereas it was only 45.3% for the conventional triptolide hydrogel. Similarly, the anti-inflammatory effect of the SLN-containing hydrogel was more than twice as much that obtained with the conventional formulation.

Besides the pharmaceutical dosage forms, a cosmetic cream formulation of Coenzyme Q10 was produced by Farboud et al. (2011). They designed this cream formulation by mixing 50% of an SLN dispersion containing Coenzyme Q10 with 50% of O/W cream and investigated the effects of lotion formulations containing pure Coenzyme Q10 and formulations with Coenzyme Q10-loaded SLNs on volunteers aged between 20 and 30. The skin hydration and elasticity evaluation performed on 25 volunteers treated with the SLN loaded lotions indicated greater skin moisture and elasticity compared to the conventional lotion. Similarly, Korkmaz et al. (2013) formulated Coenzyme Q10 loaded SLNs by a high shear homogenisation method and incorporated the SLNs into Carbopol 974P hydrogels. The gels prepared with Coenzyme Q 10-loaded SLNs were effective carrier systems for passing the active ingredient to the skin without the loss of antioxidant effects. Karavana et al. (2012) developed a buccal bioadhesive gel formulation consisting of Cyclosporine A-loaded SLNs. Invivo studies conducted on 36 rabbits revealed that the bioadhesive gel formulations containing cyclosporine A SLNssignificantly shortened the mucosal healing time, and the prepared formulation was deemed a promising system for the treatment of recurrent aphthous stomatitis.

However, the loading of SLN dispersions into the semisolid dosage form is limited and also consists of various time-consuming manufacturing steps. Additionally, incompatibility may arise between the ingredients of the hydrogel or cream formulation (e.g. emulsifying or gelling agents) and the components of an SLN dispersion (e.g. lipids or drugs) (Lippacher et al., 2001; Lippacher et al., 2002; Souto et al., 2004).

In order to prevent these problems, Lippacher et al. (2001) introduced a new one-step production method using a high-pressure homogeniser for preparing semisolid SLN formulations without any active agent. They found that the colloidal size could be preserved although the high lipid content and the semisolid consistency of the lipid dispersions. A gel-like structure of the semisolid dispersions was shown by

54

viscoelastic measurements. They concluded that the semisolid SLN dispersions developed might have a great importance for dermal applications. The researchers later showed that particle size and distributionas well as the physical state of the dispersed lipid phase have significant and important effects on the formation of semi solid gel structures (Lippacher et al., 2002).

Avery limited number of studies have been published using the one-step production of semisolid lipid nanodispersions. Teeranachaideekul et al. (2008) prepared ascorbyl palmitate-loaded semisolid nanostructured lipid carrier (NLC) dispersions using a high-pressure homogenisation technique and evaluated the physicochemical characteristics with respect to drug loading; particle size and surface charge; morphological properties; in-vitro drug release profiles; and thermal and viscoelastic behaviours of the formulations. The viscoelastic analyses showed that the developed semisolid NLC formulations had more elasticity than viscous properties, indicating a gel-like structure. In another study, Wu et al. (2010) producedsemisolid lipid nanoparticles of paclitaxel by an emulsion-solvent evaporation technique, using ethanol and acetone as organic solvents. They concluded that the developed formulation had excellent colloidal stability and high encapsulation efficiency.

In the light of these findings, semisolid SLN formulations were developed in our laboratory by a novel one-step production technique, which is a combination of high-shear homogenization and ultrasonication methods without use of organic solvents (Badilli et al., 2015). Etofenamate, a non-steroid anti-inflammatory drug that inhibits the synthesis of peripheral prostaglandins through the blockage of cyclooxygenase (COX) enzyme, was used as the active substance. Several commercial semisolid dosage forms of etofenamate for topical application are already present in the market. However, no research has been conducted related to the encapsulation of etofenamate in drug delivery systems such as SLN dispersions. We fabricated semisolid SLN formulations using Compritol 888 ATO and Precirol ATO 5 as different types of lipids. Three different lipid concentrations and two different Tween 80 concentrations were investigated as formulation parameters (Badilli et al., 2015). The codes and compositions of the semisolid SLN formulations are shown in Table 1.

Table 1. The codes and compositions of semisolid solid lipid nanoparticle (SLN) formulations.

Code	Compritol 888 ATO (%)	Precirol ATO 5 (%)	Poloxamer 188 (%)	Tween 80 (%)
C1	10	-	1.35	0.17
C2	15	-	1.35	0.17
C3	20	-	1.35	0.17
C4	10	-	1.35	0.51
C5	15	-	1.35	0.51
C6	20	-	1.35	0.51
P1	-	10	1.35	0.17
P2	-	15	1.35	0.17
P3	-	20	1.35	0.17
P4	-	10	1.35	0.51
P5	-	15	1.35	0.51
P6	-	20	1.35	0.51

In vitro characterisation of the formulations was carried out by analysing encapsulation efficiency, particle size, zeta potential and morphology (by TEM). The encapsulation efficiency of etofenamate into semisolid SLN formulations was obtained in the range of 99.64-99.98% (Figure 1). These high values for encapsulation efficiency showed the great lipid solubility of the etofenamate and also demonstrated the suitability of the Compritol and Precirol as lipid compounds for the production of the SLN formulations loaded with hydrophobic agents like etofenamate.

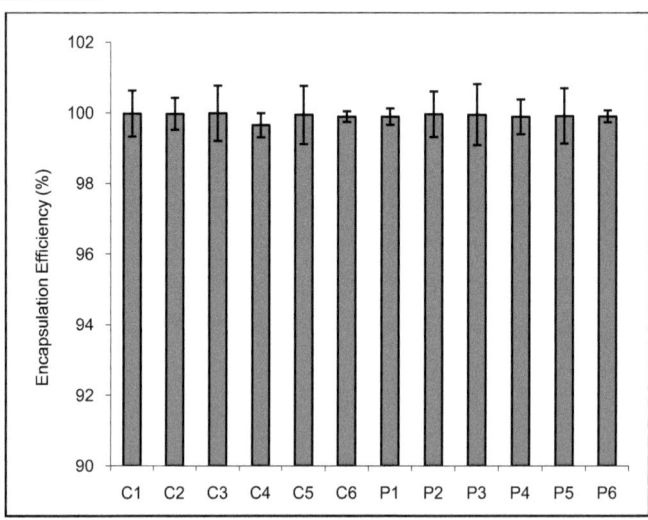

Figure 1. Encapsulation efficiency values of the semisolid solid lipid nanoparticle (SLN) formulations.

The semisolid SLN formulations have colloidal particle sizes in spite of their high lipid contents. Particle sizes and size distributions of formulations are given in Figure 2. The particle size significantly increased with the increase in the lipid concentration for both types of lipids ($p<0.05$). High lipid concentrations resulted in increasing viscosity of the dispersed phase, so larger lipid droplets formed during the emulsification process. This situation can also be explained with respect to the predisposition of lipid to coalescence at high lipid concentrations (Shah et al., 2011). When the Tween 80 concentration was enhanced from 0.17% to 0.51%, the particle sizes of formulations prepared with Compritol 888 ATO decreased for each concentration of lipid ($p<0.05$). Similar results were also obtained for the formulations prepared with Precirol ATO 5. The increase in the Tween 80 concentration resulted in a reduction in the interfacial tension between aqueous and organic phases, but was coupled with stabilisation of the newly generated surfaces and an increase in the rate of particle disintegration (Attama et al., 2007; Shah et al., 2011). The zeta potential values ranged between -31.4 mV and -41.8 mV for all formulations prepared. The zeta potential is an important parameter because it measures the stability of a colloidal system: A system with a high positive or negative value ($\pm$ 30 mV) is considered a stable formulation (Rahman et al., 2010).

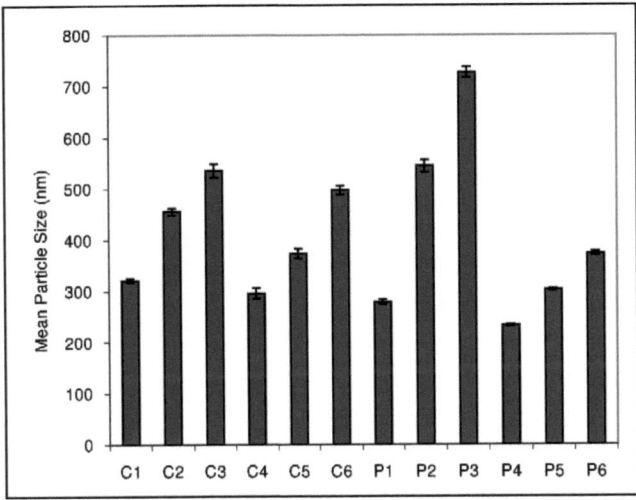

Figure 2. Mean particle sizes of semisolid solid lipid nanoparticle (SLN) formulations.

TEM images of semisolid SLN formulations are shown in Figure 3, which shows that particles of C1 and P1 coded formulations have colloidal size and spherical shape. No aggregation was observed in either of the SLN formulations.

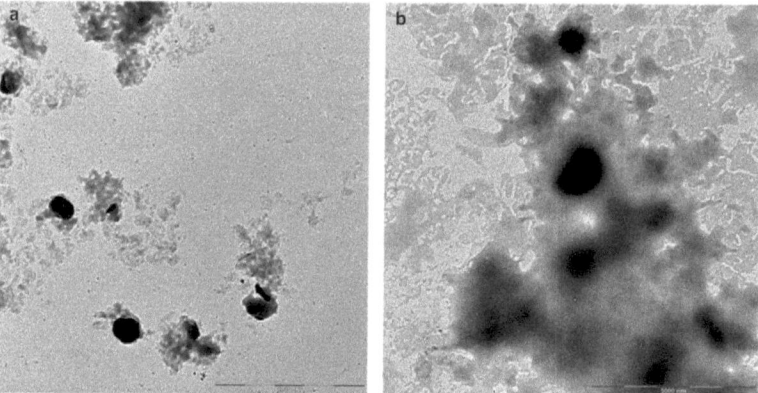

Figure 3. Transmission electron microscopy (TEM) images of C1 (a) and P1 (b) coded semisolid sold lipid nanoparticle (SLN) formulations.

The possible interactions between etofenamate and the various excipients, as well as the thermal behaviour of the lipid materials used in the semisolid SLN formulations, were investigated by differential scanning calorimetry (DSC) analysis.No interaction was observed between the active substance and the excipients. No changes appeared in the melting temperatures or the peaks of either of the lipid materials in the semisolid SLN formulations, indicating that the preparation procedure did not affect the thermal behaviour of the lipids in the formulations.

The rheological properties and in vitro drug release capabilities of the semisolid formulations were also characterised. The rheological characterisation of a semisolid system is very important since this physical parameter affects all steps of the manufacturing process and is a valuable tool in quality control of the final product. Drug release from a semisolid carrier is also influenced by the rheological behaviour.

A semisolid demonstrates both solid and liquid characteristics. Viscoelastic measurements are based on the mechanical properties of materials that exhibit both viscous properties of liquids and elastic properties of solids. Viscoelastic analysis performed by creep or oscillatory methods is particularly useful for studying the structure of semisolids. Oscillation tests are dynamic methods for determining the viscoelastic properties of the material and do not destroy the static structure, unlike continuous-shear techniques. An oscillation frequency sweep test measures the response of the tested system as a function of frequency at constant stress amplitude. It demonstrates the storage modulus, the loss modulus, and the complex viscosity (η^*). The storage modulus (G') gives information about the elastic response, while the loss modulus (G") is a measure of the viscous response (Lippacher et al., 2001; Lippacher et al., 2002; Sinko, 2011).

The oscillation frequency sweep test was performed to understand the viscoelastic behaviour of our SLN formulations. The storage modulus (G'; elastic component) was significantly higher than the loss modulus (G"; viscous component) throughout the whole frequency range for all formulations. These results confirmed that the semisolid SLN formulations had a gel-like structure and they were more elastic than viscous at the frequency range investigated. All SLN formulations showed an increment of storage modulus (G') and a decrement of loss modulus (G") with increasing frequency. On the other hand, the complex viscosity (η^*) values decreased when the frequency was increased. This behaviour is also specific for viscoelastic solids (Figure 4) (Lippacher et al., 2001; Lippacher et al., 2004).

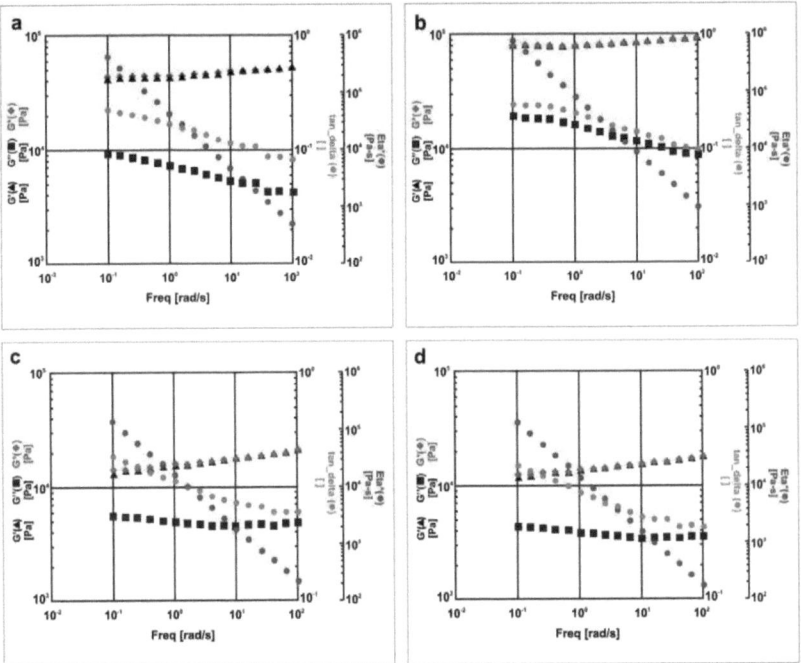

Figure 4. Oscillation frequency sweep test diagrams of C1 (a), C4 (b), P1 (c) and P4 (d) coded semisolid solid lipid nanoparticle (SLN) formulations.

In vitro etofenamate release from semisolid SLN formulations is shown in Figure 5. The release rate of etofenamate significantly increased when the lipid concentration was decreased for the formulations prepared with 0.17% Tween 80 and Compritol 888 ATO ($p<0.05$) (Figure 5a). The amount of etofenamate released at the end of the eighth hour was 153 $\mu g/cm^2$ for the formulation containing 10% lipid (C1), whereas theamountreleased from the C3 coded formulation (20% lipid) was 119 $\mu g/cm^2$. Similar release profiles were obtained for the C4, C5 and C6 coded formulations prepared using 0.51% Tween 80 and Compritol 888 ATO ($p<0.05$) (Figure 5b). When the Precirol ATO 5 formulations containing 0.17% Tween 80 were evaluated in terms of the release profiles, the highest drug release was also observed for the lipid concentration of 10% (P1) (Figure 5c). The amount of etofenamate releasedat the end of 8 h was 162 $\mu g/cm^2$, 129 $\mu g/cm^2$ and 113 $\mu g/cm^2$ for P1, P2 and P3 coded formulations, respectively ($p<0.05$). Consistent with these results, the drug release from the P4 coded formulation prepared with 10% Precirol ATO 5 was significantly faster than that from the P5 (15% lipid) and P6 (20% lipid) coded formulations ($p<0.05$) (Figure 5d). These results can all be explained by the lipid contents and particle sizes of the formulations. Decreasing lipid concentration resulted in a reduction of the viscosity and the particle size of the formulations. As a consequence, enhancement of the drug release rate was observed for the formulations with low lipid concentrations.

The storage stability studies, performed at 4°C over a six-month period, confirmed that etofenamate-loaded semisolid SLN formulations remained stable after six months of storage (Table 2). None of the investigated parameters showed any significant changes during the storage period ($P>0.05$). The encapsulation efficiency of the systems remained invariable during that time for both formulations, indicating no expulsion from the SLN particles. Storage at a temperature of 4°C was a suitable condition for the stability of semisolid SLN formulations with regards to their various physicochemical properties.

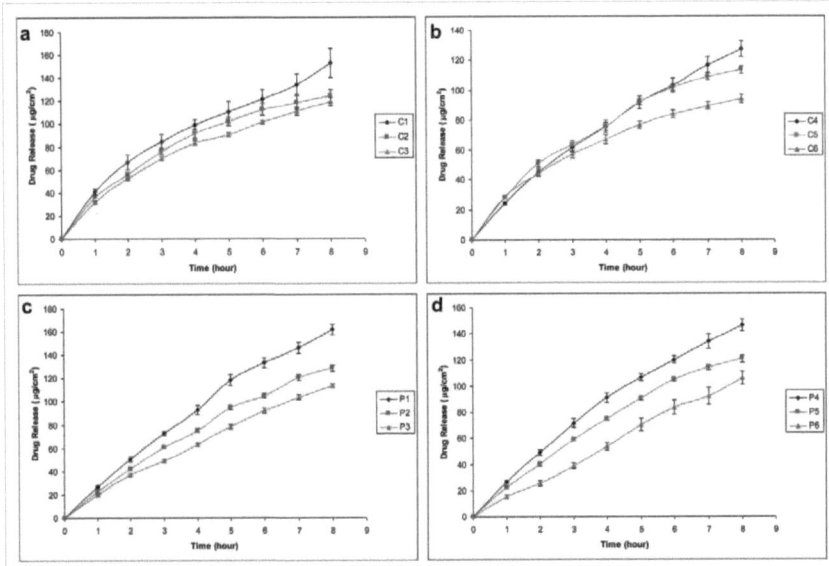

Figure 5. In vitro drug release profiles of etofenamate from semisolid solid lipid nanoparticle (SLN) formulations prepared with; a) 0.17% Tween 80 and Compritol 888 ATO, b) 0.51% Tween 80 and Compritol 888 ATO, c) 0.17% Tween 80 and Precirol ATO 5, d) 0.51% Tween 80 and Precirol ATO 5 (n=3).

Table 2. Storage stability results of the etofenamate loaded semisolid solid lipid nanoparticle (SLN) formulations (n=5).

Code	Storage period	$EE^{\#}$ (%) (Mean±$SD^{\ddagger}$)	Size (nm) (Mean ± $SD^{\ddagger}$)	PDI (Mean ± $SD^{\ddagger}$)	Zeta potential (mV) (Mean ± $SD^{\ddagger}$)
C1	1 month	99.52 ± 0.33	319.4 ± 7.2	0.307 ± 0.027	-29.9 ± 0.6
	3 months	98.26 ± 1.72	323.5 ± 3.3	0.283 ± 0.063	-31.9 ± 2.3
	6 months	99.33 ± 0.41	320.7 ± 1.8	0.270 ± 0.023	-31.5 ± 0.3
P1	1 month	98.57 ± 1.27	286.6 ± 2.7	0.362 ± 0.010	-32.9 ± 0.9
	3 months	98.91 ± 1.54	294.3 ± 1.1	0.370 ± 0.052	-33.9 ± 0.3
	6 months	98.85 ± 1.10	286.5 ± 1.7	0.382 ± 0.028	-34.1 ± 0.4

encapsulation efficiency
‡ standard deviation

The anti-inflammatory activity of the selected formulations was also evaluated. The inhibitory effects of the C1 and P1 coded semisolid SLN formulations on COX enzyme were examined to evaluate the efficacy of our formulations as potential topical treatments. The IC50 values of etofenamate in the literature were used to establish a concentration of 10^{-5} M for the study. The inhibition of COX enzyme by C1 and P1 coded semisolid SLN formulations, as well as by etofenamate in its pure form, is shown in Figure 6. The semisolid SLN formulation prepared with Compritol 888 ATO showed higher anti-inflammatory activity than the formulation containing Precirol ATO 5 or the solution of pure etofenamate.

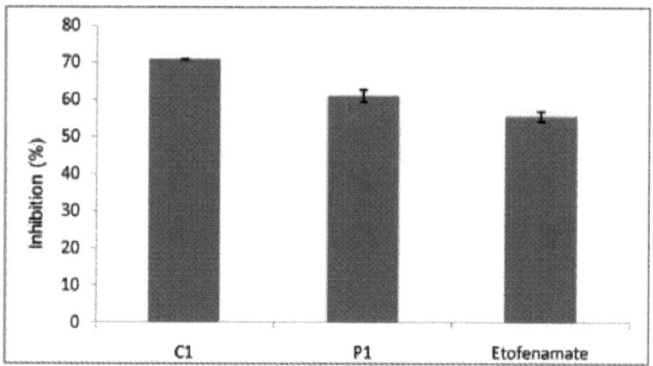

Figure 6. Anti-inflammatory activities of semisolid SLN formulations and pure etofenamate (n=3).

To the best of our knowledge, the present work is the first to report the successful preparation of etofenamate-loaded semisolid SLN formulations in a novel one-step production method, using high-shear homogenisation and ultrasonication techniques.

REFERENCES

Attama, A.A.; Schicke, B.C.; Paepenmuller, T.; Muller-Goymann, C.C. Solid lipid nanodispersions containing mixed lipid coreand a polar heterolipid: characterization. *Eur. J. Pharm. Biopharm.*, 67: 48-57, 2007.

Badilli, U., Sengel-Turk, C.T., Onay-Besikci, A., Tarimci, N. Development of etofenamate-loaded semisolid SLN dispersions and evaluation of anti-inflammatory activity for topical application. *Curr. Drug Deliv.,*12(2): 200-209, 2015.

Dingler, A., Blum, R.P., Niehus, H., Müller, R.H., Gohla, S. Solid lipid nanoparticles (SLN/Lipopearls). A pharmaceutical and cosmetic carrier for the application of vitamin E in dermal products. *J. Microencapsul.*, 16: 751-767, 1999.

Farboud, E.S., Nasrollahi, S.A., Tabbakhi, Z. Novel formulation and evaluation of a Q 10-loaded solid lipid nanoparticle cream: in vitro and in vivo studies. *Int. J. Nanomed.*, 6: 611-617, 2011.

Jenning, V., Gysler, A., Schafer-Korting, M., Gohla, S.H. Vitamin A loaded solid lipid nanoparticles for topical use: occlusive properties and drug targeting to the upper skin. *Eur. J. Pharm. Biopharm.*, 49: 211-218, 2000.

Karavana, S.Y., Gökçe, E.H., Rençber, S., Özbal, S., Pekçetin, C., Güneri, P., Ertan, G. A new approach to the treatment of recurrent aphthous stomatitis with bioadhesive gels containing cyclosporine A solid lipid nanoparticles: in vivo/in vitro examinations. *Int. J. Nanomedicine*, 7: 5693-5704, 2012.

Korkmaz, E., Gokce, E.H., Ozer, O. Development and evaluation of coenzyme Q10 loaded solid lipid nanoparticle hydrogel for enhanced dermal delivery. *Acta Pharm.*, 63: 517-529, 2013.

Lippacher, A., Müller, R.H., Mäder, K. Preparation of semisolid drug carriers for topical application based on solid lipid nanoparticles. *Int. J. Pharm.*, 214: 9-12, 2001.

Lippacher, A., Müller, R.H., Mäder, K. Semisolid SLN^{TM} dispersions for topical application: influence of formulation and production parameters on viscoelastic properties. *Eur. J. Pharm. Biopharm.*, 53: 155-160, 2002.

Lippacher, A.; Muller, R.H.; Mader, K. Liquid and semisolid SLN™ dispersions for topical application: rheological characterization. *Eur. J. Pharm. Biopharm.*, 58: 561-567, 2004.

Mei, Z., Wu, Q., Hu, S., Li, X., Yang, X. Triptolide loaded solid lipid nanoparticle hydrogel for topical application. *Drug Development and Industrial Pharmacy*, 31: 161–168, 2005.

Prow, T.W.; Grice, J.E.; Lin, L.L.; Faye, R.; Butler, M.; Becker, W.; Wurm, E.M.T.; Yoong, C.; Robertson, T.A.; Soyer, H.P.; Roberts, M.S. Nanoparticles and microparticles for skin drug delivery. *Adv. Drug Del. Rev.*, 63: 470-491, 2011.

Rahman, Z.; Zidan, A.S.; Khan, M.A. Non-destructive methods of characterization of risperidone solid lipid nanoparticles. *Eur. J. Pharm. Biopharm.*, 76: 127-137, 2010.

Santos Maia, C., Mehnert, W., Schaller, M., Korting, H.C., Gysler, A., Haberland, A., Schäfer-Korting, M. Drug targeting by solid lipid nanoparticles for dermal use. *Journal of Drug Targeting*, 10(6): 489-495, 2002.

Schafer-Korting, M.; Mehnert, W.; Korting, H.C. Lipid nanoparticles for improved topical application of drugs for skin diseases. *Adv. Drug Del. Rev.*, 59: 427-443, 2007.

Shah, M.; Chuttani, K.; Mishra, A.K.; Pathak, K. Oral solid compritol 888 ATO nanosuspension of simvastatin: optimization and biodistribution studies. *Drug Dev. Ind. Pharm.*, 37: 526-537, 2011.

Sinko, P.J. Martin's Physical Pharmacy and Pharmaceutical Sciences: Physical, Chemical and Biopharmaceutical Principles in the Pharmaceutical Sciences, 6th ed.; Walters Kluwer − Lippincott Williams & Wilkins: Philadelphia, 469-491, 2011.

Souto, E.B., Wissing, S.A., Barbosa, C.M., Müller, R.H. Evaluation of the physical stability of SLN and NLC before and after incorporation into hydrogel formulations. *Eur. J. Pharm. Biopharm.*, 8: 83-90, 2004.

Souto, E.B., Almeida, A.J.; Muller, R.H. Lipid nanoparticles (SLN®, NLC®) for cutaneous drug delivery: structure, protection and skin effects. *J. Biomed. Nanotechnol.*, 3: 317-331, 2007.

Teeranachaideekul, V.; Souto, E.B.; Müller, R.H.; Junyaprasert, V.B. Physicochemical characterization and in vitro release studies of ascorbyl palmitate-loaded semi-solid nanostructured lipid carriers (NLC gels). *J. Microencapsul.*, 25: 111-120, 2008.

Wu, L., Tang, C., Yin, C. Preparation and characterization of paclitaxel delivery system based on semi-solid lipid nanoparticles coated with poly(ethylene glycol). *Pharmazie*, 65: 493-499, 2010.

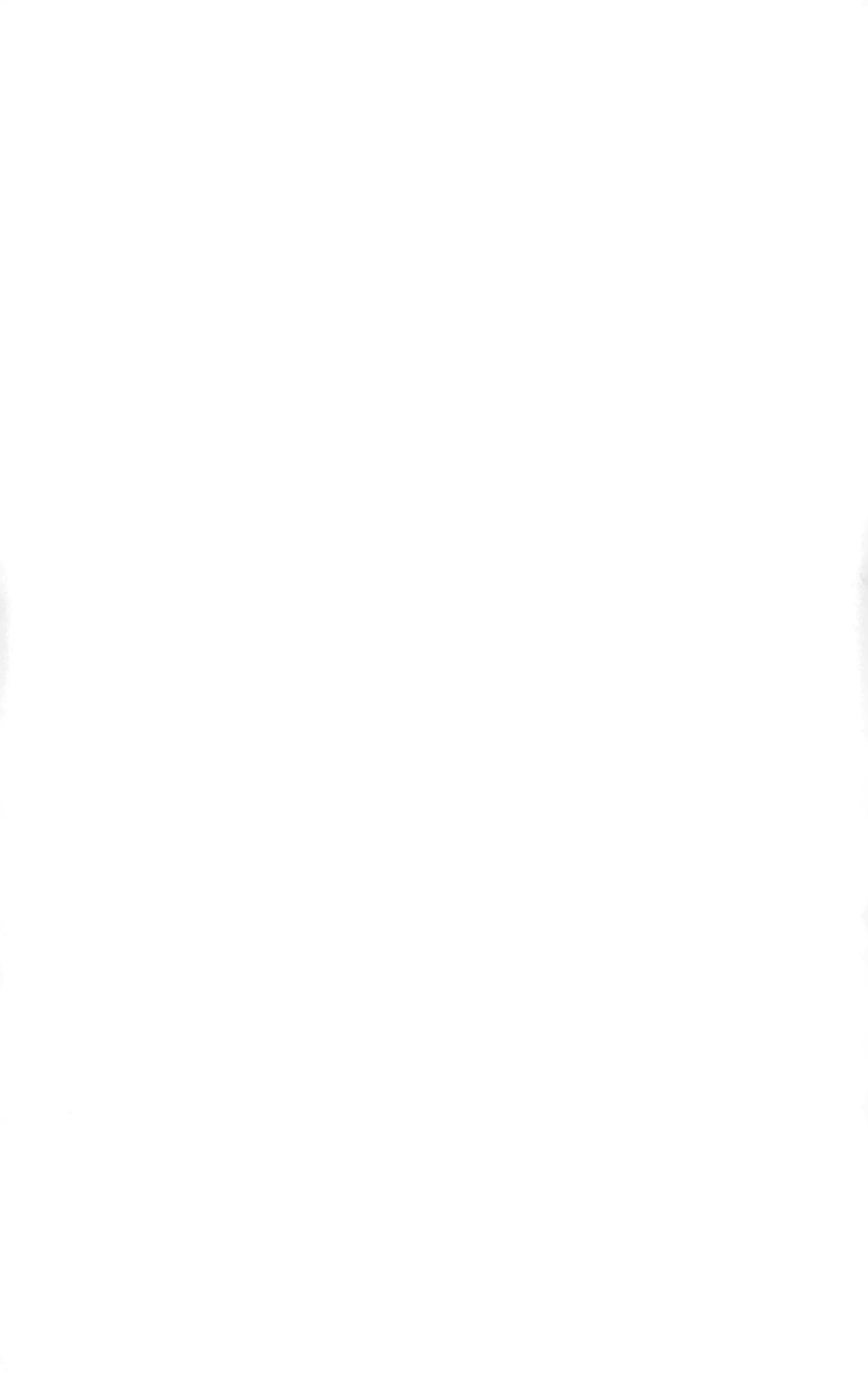

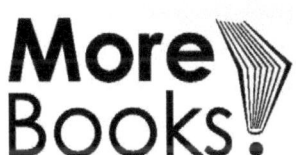
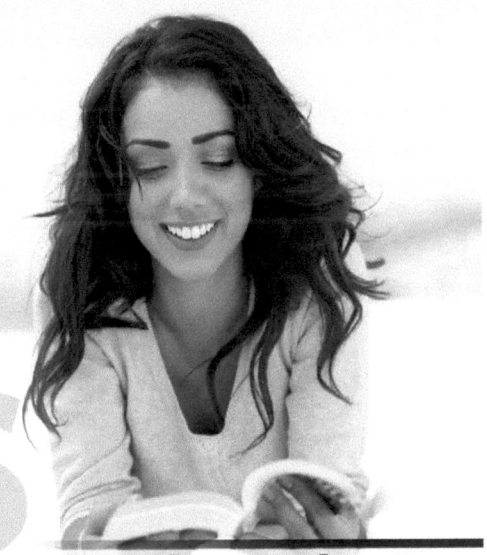
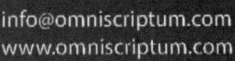
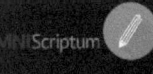

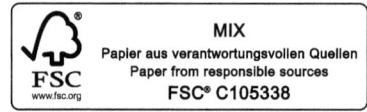

Printed by Books on Demand GmbH, Norderstedt / Germany